Oliver Kretz, Ketan Patel

Sobotta

Anatomy Coloring Book

Oliver Kretz, Ketan Patel

Sobotta

Anatomy Coloring Book

With 160 illustrations

ELSEVIER

Elsevier GmbH, Hackerbrücke 6, 80335 München, Deutschland
Please send your feedback and your suggestions to books.cs.muc@elsevier.com

Sobotta Anatomy Coloring Book
© Elsevier GmbH, Germany, 2019, All rights reserved.
ISBN 978-0-7020-5278-1

This translation of Sobotta Malbuch Anatomie, 4th edition, by Marieke O'Connor was undertaken by Elsevier GmbH.

Disclaimer

The translation has been undertaken by Elsevier GmbH at its sole responsibility. Practitioners and researchers must always rely on their own experience and knowledge in evaluating and using any information, methods, compounds or experiments described herein. Because of rapid advances in the medical sciences, in particular, independent verification of diagnoses and drug dosages should be made. To the fullest extent of the law, no responsibility is assumed by Elsevier, authors, editors or contributors in relation to the translation or for any injury and/or damage to persons or property as a matter of products liability, negligence or otherwise, or from any use or operation of any methods, products, instructions, or ideas contained in the material herein.

Bibliographic information published by the Deutsche Nationalbibliothek

The Deutsche Nationalbibliothek lists this publication in the Deutsche Nationalbibliografie; detailed bibliographic data are available on the Internet at http://www.d-nb.de.

19 20 21 22 23   5 4 3 2 1

Aquisition editior: Dr. Katja Weimann, München
Project management: Christine Kosel, München
Translation: Marieke O'Connor, Oxford/UK
Typesetting: abavo GmbH, Buchloe
Printed and bound by: Drukarnia Dimograf Sp z o.o., Bielsko-Biała/Polen
Illustrations: Andreas Dietz, Konstanz: 2.13, 2.14, 3.3, 3.4, 3.5, 3.14, 3.15, 5.4, 5.5, 5.9, 9.4, 9.6, 9.7, 9.13, 9.14, 9.24;
              Holger Keller, Freiburg: all other illustrations apart from those listed above
Cover illustration: Andreas Dietz, Konstanz
Cover design: SpieszDesign, Neu-Ulm

Current information by **www.elsevier.com**

Preface

An exact knowledge of macroscopic anatomy is the basis of medical training and is required for all medical practice. This applies to the physical examination of the patient, the assessment of diagnostic images and, needless to say, all medical procedures.

To understand complex topographical relationships, a good sense of spatial awareness is essential. Learning and understanding the positional relationships of anatomical structures by extension is best done through practical work in a gross anatomy class. Because this is only available to a limited extent in an educational capacity, one needs anatomical textbooks with good illustrative material. Furthermore, many students draw and annotate their own sketches of the anatomic structures in these textbooks and atlases. This conforms to learning theories whereby complex learning content is more easily remembered when it is actively reproduced.

On the basis of this rationale, we have developed a coloring book of anatomy, presenting those who are less artistically gifted with a model of the important and topographically complex areas of the body to color in and get to know in a more playful way.

The *Sobotta Coloring Book* is directed at students of medicine, students in healthcare professions, as well as at all those interested in human anatomy.

The **illustrations** of this coloring book have been taken from the Sobotta Atlas of Human Anatomy, which has accompanied generations of students as the standard reference in the course of their studies. Further illustrations can therefore easily be accessed and used as reference while working on the Coloring Book.

The illustrations are supplemented with **teaching material**, containing all the basic information in a precise and easily understood style, systematically and interactively guiding the reader through the illustrations. The teaching material also contains a **description for each illustration** as well as the most important **facts relevant for tests and examinations** for those areas of the body that are represented. The main points are also highlighted in an additional **Note** for each theme, and **Clinical remarks** are made about individual cases, providing interest but also acting as an aide-memoire to the student.

How to use this book

The illustrations and text in the Coloring Book have been divided into chapters according to the individual areas and organs of the body and those parts that belong to them. The illustrated pages are presented as black and white picture outlines, to be colored using colored pencils or crayons. The choice of color is not stipulated, but we recommend using similar colors to those used in standard anatomical atlases and textbooks (arteries: red; veins: blue; nerves: yellow; lymph vessels: green; muscles: red brown, etc.). The structures of the illustrated pages are numbered consecutively and can be labelled by students themselves in a self-imposed quiz.

The corresponding page with text gives a detailed description of the illustration, in which all numbered structures are explained. The text can be read before coloring the picture or can be read as a 'solution' after doing the quiz-style labels. Moreover, the text briefly gives the most important facts about the body area shown in the illustration.

The Coloring Book contains important and topographically complex body areas. To master anatomy completely and systematically, we refer students to exhaustive anatomy textbooks such as the Sobotta textbooks or the 'Benninghoff'. Critical comments and recommendations for improving this book are very welcome.

Authors

PD Dr. med. Oliver Kretz holds a habilitation in Anatomy. He currently works as lab head in the field of kidney research at the III. Department of Medicine, University Medical Center Hamburg-Eppendorf, Hamburg, Germany.
https://www.tbhuber.org/team-hamburg/laboratory-head-em-oliver-kretz-md-pd

Prof. Dr Ketan Patel is an embryologist with a special interest in the development of the musculature. He is head of the Molecular Medicine Group at the University of Reading, UK where is he is the Professor of Developmental Biology and Regenerative Medicine.
http://www.reading.ac.uk/biologicalsciences/about/staff/ketan-patel.aspx

Acknowledgements

We are particularly grateful to Mr Holger Keller, Freiburg and Dr. Andreas Dietz, Konstanz, who with great creativity and sense of commitment prepared the visually appealing and anatomically exact illustrations which bring this book alive. Additionally we would like to thank the copy-editing staff and production department at the publisher Urban & Fischer for an amicable and constructive working environment. We would also like to thank Oliver's former boss and teacher, Prof. Dr. R. Bock, Homburg/Saar, for a critical review of the texts. We wish all readers much success and joy in using this book.

Hamburg und Reading, January 2019
Oliver Kretz & Ketan Patel

General directional and positional terms of the body

The following terms describe the position of organs and parts of the body in relation to each other, irrespective of the position of the body (e.g. supine or upright) or direction and position of the limbs. These terms are relevant not only for human anatomy but also for clinical medicine and comparative anatomy.

General terms

anterior – posterior = in front – behind (e.g. Arteriae tibiales anterior and posterior)

ventralis – dorsalis = towards the stomach – towards the back

superior – inferior = above – below (e.g. Conchae nasales superior and inferior)

cranialis – caudalis = towards the head – towards the tail

dexter – sinister = right – left (e.g. Arteriae iliacae communes dextra and sinistra)

internus – externus = internal – external

superficialis – profundus = superfical – deep (e.g. Musculi flexores digitorum superficialis and profundus)

medius, intermedius = located between two other structures (e.g. the Concha nasalis media lies between the Concha nasalis superior and inferior.)

medianus = located in the midline (e.g. Fissura mediana anterior of the spinal cord; the median plane is a sagittal plane which divides the body into an identical right and left half).

medialis – lateralis = located near the midline, located away from the midline of the body (e.g. Fossae inguinales medialis and lateralis)

frontalis = located in a frontal plane, but also towards the front (e.g. Processus frontalis of the maxilla)

longitudinalis = parallel to the longitudinal axis (e.g. Musculus longitudinalis superior of the tongue)

sagittalis = located in a sagittal plane

transversalis = located in a transverse plane

transversus = running in a transverse direction (e.g. Processus transversus of the thoracic vertebra)

Terms of direction and position for the limbs

proximalis – distalis = located towards or away from the attached end of a limb or the origin of a structure (e.g. Articulationes radioulnares proximalis and distalis)

for the upper limb:
radialis – ulnaris = located on the radial side – located on the ulnar side (e.g. Arteriae radialis and ulnaris)

for the hand:
palmaris – dorsalis = located towards the palm of the hand – located towards the back of the hand (e.g. Aponeurosis palmaris, Musculus interosseus dorsalis)

for the lower limb:
tibialis – fibularis = located on the tibial side – located on the fibular side (e.g. Arteria tibialis anterior)

for the foot:
plantaris – dorsalis = located towards the sole of the foot – located towards the back of the foot (e.g. Arteriae plantares lateralis and medialis, Arteria dorsalis pedis)

Abbreviations

A.; Aa.	=	Arteria; Arteriae (plural)
Art.	=	Articulatio
Gl.; Gll.	=	Glandula; Glandulae (plural)
Lig.; Ligg.	=	Ligamentum; Ligamenta (plural)
M.; Mm.	=	Musculus; Musculi (plural)
N.; Nn.	=	Nervus; Nervi (plural)
Ncl.; Ncll.	=	Nucleus; Nuclei (plural)
Proc.; Procc.	=	Processus; Processus (plural)
R.; Rr.	=	Ramus; Rami (plural)
V.; Vv.	=	Vena; Venae (plural)

Content

1.1 Superficial, extrinsic muscles of the back

The muscles of the back comprise two groups with different origins:

- The **superficial back muscles** originate mostly from insertion on the upper extremity and migrate **secondarily** towards the back during development.
- The **deep back muscles** originate **autochthonously (originate where found)** from the dorsal myotomes (➤ Chap. 1.2).

Extrinsic (superficial) muscles These muscles essentially originate from the spine and/or the head and insert at the upper extremity. The following muscle groups are differentiated:

- suprascapular group
- scapulohumeral group
- serratus posterior group

Suprascapular group This group consists of M. trapezius, the Mm. rhomboidei and the M. levator scapulae. The Mm. rhomboidei and the M. levator scapulae are only visible after the M. trapezius has been removed.

The **M. trapezius (1a–d)** originates from the Linea nuchalis superior, from the nuchal ligament as well as from the spinous processes of the thoracic vertebrae. In the centre of both the muscles (approx. at the level of the 7th cervical vertebra) there is a rhomboid **tendinous zone or mirror (1d)**. The fibres of the M. trapezius converge laterally and attach to the clavicula, the acromion and the Spina scapulae. Corresponding to the wide-ranging origin and the convergence of the muscle fibres towards the insertion point, one can differentiate a **Pars descendens (1a)**, a **Pars horizontalis (1b)** and a **Pars ascendens (1c)**. The M. trapezius pulls the scapula downwards, upwards or medially. If the scapula is the Punctum fixum, the Pars descendens **(1a)** sets the head into the neck. The M. trapezius is innervated by the N. accessorius (N. XI) and by branches from the Plexus cervicalis.

The **Mm. rhomboidei major (2)** and **minor (3)** originate from the spinous processes of the lower cervical and upper thoracic vertebrae and run towards the medial margin of the scapula. They fix the scapula at the trunk and run medially upwards.

The **M. levator scapulae (4)** originates from the transverse processes of the first four cervical vertebrae and runs to the Angulus superior of the scapula. It lifts this upwards and simultaneously causes a turning of the shoulder blade so that the Angulus inferior moves closer to the spine. The Mm. rhomboidei and the levator scapulae are innervated by the N. dorsalis scapulae

from the Plexus brachialis. Turning and shifting the scapula by using the different extrinsic back muscles facilitates a greater range of movement in the upper extremity.

Scapulohumeral group This group only consists of the **M. latissimus dorsi (5)**. It originates from the spinous processes of the lower thoracic and all the lumbar vertebrae as well as from the **Fascia thoracolumbalis (6)**. The fibres of the M. latissimus dorsi converge in a spiral shape and insert at the Crista tuberculi minoris of the humerus. The M. latissimus dorsi retroverts, adducts and rotates inwards in the shoulder joint and is innervated by the N. thoracodorsalis from the Plexus brachialis.

Serratus posterior muscle group The **M. serratus posterior inferior (7)** and the **M. serratus posterior superior** (not shown) belong to this group. The M. serratus posterior superior lifts the 2nd–5th ribs and is innervated by anterior branches from the C6–C8. The M. serratus posterior inferior draws the ribs downwards and is innervated by anterior branches from the Th12–L2.

> **Note**
>
> The **superficial back muscles** essentially come from the insertion point on the upper extremity. In this way many muscles of this group are innervated by the nerves of the Plexus brachialis, therefore from the **Rr. anteriores of the spinal nerves C5–Th1**. The **M. trapezius** is an exception here: it is innervated by the **N. accessorius**.

> **Clinical remarks**
>
> With **paralysis of the Mm. rhomboidei,** the Angulus inferior of the Scapula protrudes from the trunk (Scapula alata).

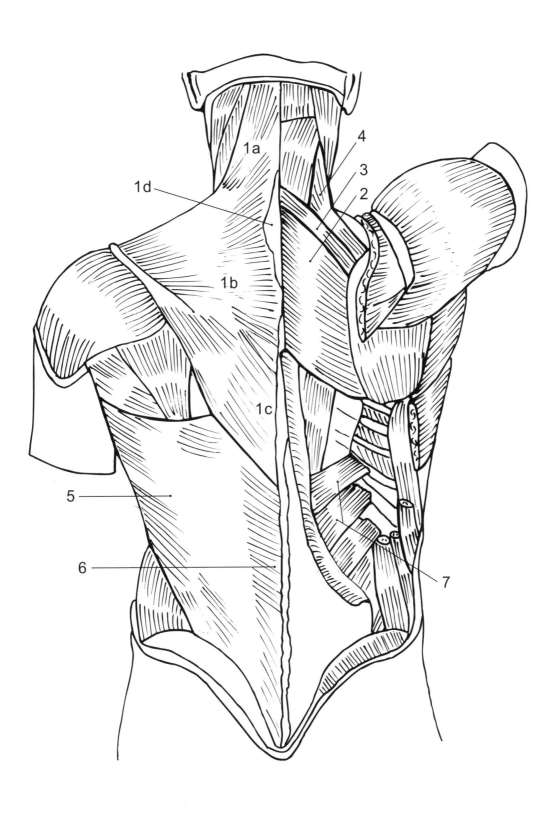

Abb. 1.1

3

1.2 Deep muscles of the back

The deep muscles of the back originate autochthonously from the dorsal myotomes and are thereby innervated by the Rr. posteriores of the spinal nerves. As a whole, the autochthonous back muscles, which consist of numerous single muscles, are also known as **M. erector spinae**. They form two muscle strands lateral of the spinous processes of the vertebrae:

- the more superficial **lateral tract** and
- the deeper **medial tract**.

Lateral tract The most important muscles of the tract are:

- the **M. iliocostalis (1)**
- the **M. longissimus (2a–c)**
- the **Mm. splenii**

The **M. iliocostalis (1)** belongs to the sacrospinal system due to its course. It originates at different levels from the Ala ossis ilium as well as from the lower and upper ribs, runs upwards and attaches in turn to the ribs or the transverse processes of the cervical vertebrae. Thereby a lumbar, thoracic and cervical part of the muscle can be differentiated. On the right side of the illustration, the overlapping origins and insertions of the **M. iliocostalis (Ia and Ib)** are schematically depicted. A one-sided contraction of the muscles leads to an inclination to the side, a bilateral contraction leads to stretching of the spine.

The **M. longissimus (2a–c)** is located somewhat further medially. It is also seen as part of the sacrospinal system and consists of a thoracic, cervical and head part. The **M. longissimus thoracis (2a)** originates from the Os sacrum and inserts at numerous points into the Procc. accessorii of the lumbar vertebrae, the transverse processes of the thoracic vertebrae and the ribs. The **M. longissimus cervicis (2b)** originates from the transverse processes of the thoracic vertebrae and runs to the transverse processes of the cervical vertebrae. The **M. longissimus capitis (2c)** runs from the transverse processes of the lower cervical and upper thoracic vertebrae to Proc. mastoideus. The location of the different origin points and insertion points of the **M. longissimus (IIa–c)** is depicted schematically on the right hand side of the illustration. The function of the M. longissimus corresponds broadly to that of the M. iliocostalis. The M. longissimus capitis also inclines the head and turns it to the same side.

The **Mm. splenii** belong to the **spinotransversal system**. These proceed from the spinous processes to the transverse processes of the cranially located vertebrae and to the back of the head. Due to its orientation, a one-sided contraction, results in a turning of the spine and/or the head on the same side.

Medial tract This tract lies in the groove between the spinous and transverse processes of the vertebra. Based on the course of the muscles, we can differentiate between the **spinal** and the **transversospinal** system:

The **M. spinalis (3)** can be seen on the **spinal system**. It occurs mostly in the thoracic area and runs from the spinous process to the spinous process, skipping numerous segments. The Mm. interspinales also belongs to the spinal system, only straddling one segment. Due to its course, the spinal system induces predominantly a stretching of the spine.

The **transversospinal system** runs from transverse processes (4) to spinous processes (5) of vertebrae lying more cranially. The **Mm. rotatores breves (6)** and **longi (7)** are the shortest muscles of this group. They each straddle one or two segments. The **Mm. multifidi** also belong to the **transversospinal system**. They are of particularly evident in the lumbar area, straddling 3–5 vertebrae (not shown). **M. semispinalis**, also belongs to this group and spans 4–6 segments and divides into the thoracic, cervical and head parts. The **Mm. semispinales thoracis (8a)** and **capitis (8b)** can be seen on the illustration. The transversospinal system stretches the spine and inclines to the side with a one-sided action. Additionally, with a one-sided action, the spine and/or the head are turned to the opposite side.

> **Note**
>
> The **autochthonous muscles of the back** originate from dorsal myotomes and are innervated by the **Rr. posteriores of the spinal nerves (C1–S1)**.

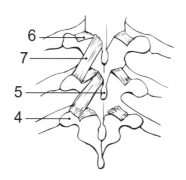

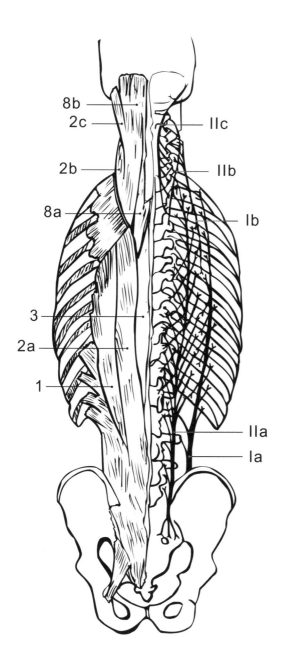

Abb. 1.2

1.3 Short muscles of the neck and Trigonum arteriae vertebralis

Short muscles of the neck   When dissecting the M. trapezius in the same way as the Mm. splenius and semispinalis capitis in the area of the neck, one exposes the deep muscles of the neck. These are the autochtonous muscles of the neck, which span the lower and upper head joint. In the lower head joint, between the atlas and the axis, turning movements of the head, amongst others, can be conducted around a vertical axis (through the dens axis). In the upper head joint between the condyles of the Os occipitale and the Facies articulares superiores of the atlas, one can incline the head to the side and nod. The following belong to the deep muscles of the neck:

- the **M. rectus capitis posterior major (1)**
- the **M. rectus capitis posterior minor (2)**
- the **M. obliquus capitis superior (3)**
- the **M. obliquus capitis inferior (4)**

The **M. rectus capitis posterior major (1)** originates from the **spinous process of the axis (5)** and runs upwards to the Linea nuchalis inferior.

Partially covered by it, the **M. rectus capitis posterior minor (2)** runs from the **Tuberculum posterius of the atlas (6a)** upwards and adheres a little caudally of the Linea nuchalis inferior to the occiput. With bilateral activity, both muscles effect a dorsal flexion of the head and with unilateral activity they effect a torsion on the same side.

The **M. obliquus capitis superior (3)** originates from the **transverse process of the atlas (6b)**. It runs diagonally upwards and attaches laterally from the M. rectus capitis posterior major onto the Squama occipitalis. It results in a dorsal extension in the upper head joint as well as with a unilateral movement in an inclination on the side of the head.

The **M. obliquus capitis inferior (4)** connects the **spinous process of the axis (5)** with the **transverse process of the atlas (6b)**. A unilateral contraction of the muscle induces a torsion to the same side in the lower head joint.

Trigonum arteriae vertebralis   The Mm. obliqui capitis superior (3) and inferior (4) as well as the M. rectus capitis posterior major (1) confine the Trigonum arteriae vertebralis. It derives its name from the **A. vertebralis (7)**, which runs in the depths of the triangle from lateral to medial on the **Arcus atlantis (arch of the atlas, 6c)** to the Foramen magnum of the Os occipitale.

The **N. suboccipitalis (8)** is the most important nerve in the Trigonum arteriae vertebralis. It represents the R. posterior of the spinal nerve C1 and innervates the short muscles of the neck. The N. suboccipitalis does not have a cutaneous branch, which means that the skin on the occiput is innervated by the cutaneous branch from the Rr. posteriores of the spinal nerve C2. The **N. occipitalis major (9)** is the corresponding nerve, penetrating the short muscles of the neck and the M. semispinalis capitis, ultimately reaching the surface at the insertion point of the M. trapezius. Caudally, the next adjoining nerve is the **N. occipitalis tertius (10)**, which emerges from the R. posterior of the third cervical spinal nerve.

Note

The **Trigonum arteriae vertebralis** is confined by the Mm. rectus capitis posterior major, obliquus capitis superior and obliquus capitis inferior. The **A. vertebralis** and the **N. suboccipitalis** are also located here.

The Nn. suboccipitalis, occipitalis major and occipitalis tertius originate from the **Rr. posteriores of the first three cervical spinal nerves**. In contrast, the N. occipitalis minor, which also runs occipitally, originates from the Plexus cervicalis and thereby from the **Rr. anteriores** (C2) of the cervical spinal nerves.

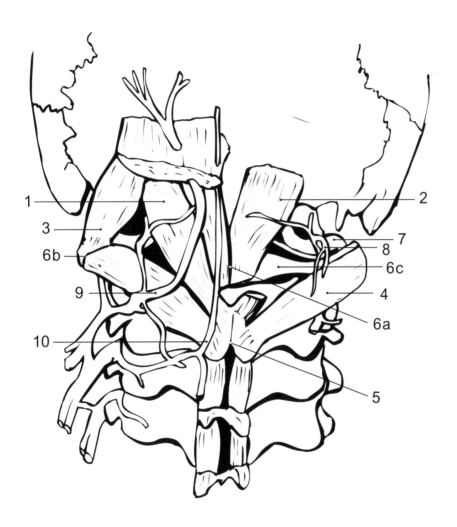

1 ——
3 —
6b —
9 —
10 —

2 ——
7
8
6c
4
6a
5

Abb. 1.3

2.1 Shoulder joint

Structure   The shoulder joint is a ball joint with an exceptional range of movement.

The **Cavitas glenoidalis (1)** of the **scapula (2)** forms the bony socket, which is augmented by a fibrous cartilaginous ring, the **Labrum glenoidale (3)**. Only approx. one-third of the **humeral head (Caput humeri, 4)** is enclosed by the Labrum glenoidale. The roof of the shoulder joint is formed by the **acromion (5)** and the **Lig. coracoacromiale (7)** which runs between it and the **Proc. coracoideus (6)**. These structures serve the humerus as an abutment in quadrupedal walking. They nevertheless also prevent mobility of the humerus and therefore need to be twisted out of the way, for example when elevating the arms while simultaneously moving the scapula. Because the humeral head moves against the acromion and the Lig. coracoacromiale, a bursa, the **Bursa subacromialis (8),** is found at this pressure and friction point.

The **articular capsule (9)** of the shoulder joint is lax and can envelop the humeral head twice over. Hereby a fold, the **Recessus axillaris (10)**, is created. The **Lig. coracohumerale (11)**, which runs from the Proc. coracoideus to the Tuberculum majus of the humerus, is the only ligament supporting the capsule. The small socket, the lax articular capsule and the barely visible ligamentous support mean that the shoulder joint must be steered muscularly through the **rotator cuff** (➤ Chap. 2.2).

The **tendon of the long head of the biceps (M. biceps brachii, Caput longum, Tendo, 12)** runs through the articular capsule of the shoulder joint und inserts – partially via the **Labrum glenoidale (3)** – at the Tuberculum supraglenoidale. The Caput longum of the **M. triceps brachii (13)** at the Tuberculum infraglenoidale attaches to the outside of the articular capsule of the shoulder.

Note

The shoulder joint is a **ball joint,** in which the humeral head and the Cavitas glenoidalis of scapula articulate with each other. It is strengthened via the muscles of the rotator cuff.

Clinical remarks

The structure of the shoulder joint and its muscular support provide the arm with great gripping possibilities. But the risk of a **dislocated shoulder** is increased. The dislocation can be caused by a trauma or through a habitual movement of the shoulder joint. **Habitual dislocations** are often caused by injuries to the Labrum glenoidale. The most common shoulder dislocation is the **Luxatio subcoracoidea,** whereby the humeral head ends up underneath the Proc. coracoideus.

Lengthy immobilisation of the shoulder joint leads to a contraction of the shoulder muscle and eventually to restricted movement.

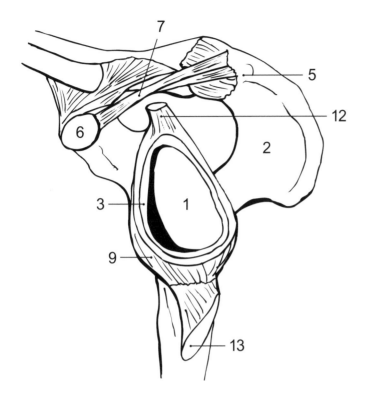

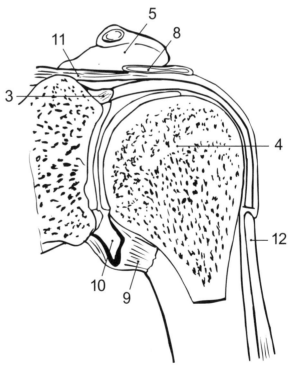

Abb. 2.1

2.2 Muscles of the shoulder

Rotator cuff The shoulder joint is supported by the muscle tendons of the rotators (the M. supraspinatus, M. infraspinatus, M. subscapularis and M. teres minor). They run cranially, ventrally and dorsally of the joint capsule, partially fusing with it and thereby support the humeral head in the joint socket. A weak spot on the caudal region remains on the joint capsule.

- **M. infraspinatus**
  The **M. infraspinatus (1)** originates from the Fossa infraspinata of the scapula. Its tendon runs dorsally around the humeral head to the Tuberculum majus of the humerus. The M. infraspinatus is innervated by the N. suprascapularis. It allows the arm to rotate outwards.

- **M. teres major**
  The **M. teres major (2)** originates from the Angulus inferior of the scapula. It then runs alongside the **M. latissimus dorsi (3)** to the Crista tuberculi minoris. The M. teres major allows the shoulder joint to rotate inwards. As with the M. latissimus dorsi the M. teres is innervated by the N. thoracodorsalis.

- **M. teres minor**
  The **M. teres minor (4)** originates from the Margo lateralis of the scapula, runs dorsally around the humeral head and inserts at the Tuberculum majus. The M. teres minor allows the arm to rotate outwards. It is innervated by the N. axillaris.

- **M. supraspinatus**
  The **M. supraspinatus (5)** originates from the Fossa supraspinata of the scapula. Its tendon runs between the acromion and the humeral head to the Tuberculum majus of the humerus. Between the tendon and the acromion is the Bursa subacromialis (➤ Chap. 2.1), which lessens the friction of the tendon when moving. The M. supraspinatus is innervated by the N. suprascapularis. It abducts the arm and additionally rotates it outwards weakly.

- **M. subscapularis**
  The **M. subscapularis (6)** originates from the Fossa subscapularis and runs ventrally of the humeral head to the Tuberculum minus. It is innervated by the N. subscapularis. The M. subscapularis rotates the arm inwards.

- **M. deltoideus**
  The **M. deltoideus (7)** originates from the **clavicula (8)**, the **acromion** and the **Spina scapulae (9)**. It covers the rounded contour of the shoulder and inserts at the **humerus (10)** at the Tuberositas deltoidea. The M. deltoideus is innervated by the N. axillaris. It abducts or elevates the arm.

Armpits The **Mm. teres major (2)** and **teres minor (4)** delineate a triangle together with the **humerus (10)**. Via this triangle the **Caput longum of the M. triceps brachii (11)** runs in the direction of the Tuberculum infraglenoidale (➤ Chap. 2.1). Thereby a triangular **medial (12)** and a square **lateral (13) armpit** is formed. The A. and V. circumflexa scapulae are in the medial armpit and the N. axillaris and die A. and V. circumflexa humeri posterior are in the lateral.

Clinical remarks

Pain and restriction of movement which accompany degenerative changes in the area of the Bursa subacromialis and the tendons of the rotator cuff (especially of the M. supraspinatus), are described as **Periarthropathia humeroscapularis**.

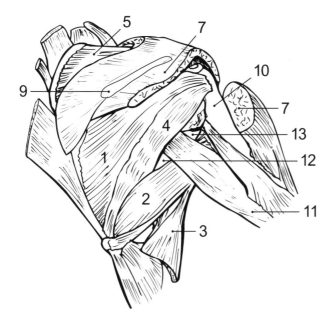

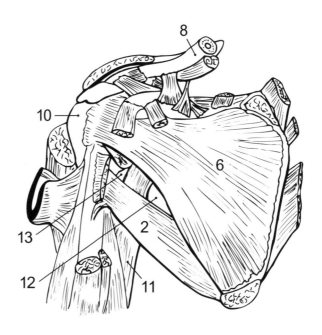

Abb. 2.2

2.3 Muscles of the upper arm

The muscles of the upper arm are divided into the:
- extensors (extending)
- flexors (flexing)

Extensors
- **M. triceps brachii**

  The **M. triceps brachii (1a–c)** is a muscle with three heads. Its **Caput longum (1a)** originates from the Tuberculum infraglenoidale of the Scapula, runs to the upper arm between the M. teres major and the M. teres minor and thereby forms a part of the boundary of the armpits. The Caput longum inserts with the terminal tendons into both the other heads on the **olecranon (2)**. Because it originates at the scapula, the Caput longum also operates the shoulder joint by making it retrovert weakly. The **Caput mediale (1b)** originates from the dorsal side of the humerus, distal of the Sulcus nervi radialis and from the Septum intermusculare mediale. The **Caput laterale (1c)** originates proximally of the Sulcus nervi radialis up to the Tuberculum majus. The three heads of the M. triceps brachii are innervated by the N. radialis.

- **M. anconeus**

  The **M. anconeus** (not shown) runs from the Epicondylus lateralis of the humerus to the olecranon and to the proximal ulna. It represents a separation of the Caput mediale from the M. triceps brachii and is innervated by the N. radialis.

Flexors
- **M. biceps brachii**

  The **Caput longum of the M. biceps brachii (3a)** originates from the Tuberculum supraglenoidale of the scapula. Its tendon runs through the shoulder joint (➤ Chap. 2.1) and leaves through the Sulcus intertubercularis. The **Caput breve of the M. biceps brachii (3b)** originates from the Proc. coracoideus of the scapula. Both heads unite and their **main tendon (3c)** attaches itself to the Tuberositas radii. This superficial adjoining tendon radiates as the **Aponeurosis musculi bicipitis brachii (3d)** into the antebrachial fascia. Both heads flex in the elbow joint and supinate the forearm. The Caput longum abducts and rotates inwards, the Caput breve adducts and rotates inwards in the shoulder joint. The M. biceps brachii is innervated by the N. musculocutaneus.

- **M. brachialis**

  The **M. brachialis (4)** originates from the front surface of the humerus and inserts at the Tuberositas ulnae. It flexes in the humeroulnar joint and is innervated by the N. musculocutaneus.

- **M. coracobrachialis**

  The **M. coracobrachialis (5)** orginates like the Caput breve of the M. biceps brachii from the Proc. coracoideus of the scapula and inserts on the medial side of the humerus, distal of the Crista tuberculi minoris. The M. coracobrachialis weakly anteverts and adducts the shoulder joint. It is penetrated and also innervated by the N. musculocutaneus.

> **Note**
>
> **Innervation of the muscles of the upper arm**
> Flexors → N. musculocutaneus
> Extensors → N. radialis

> **Clinical remarks**
>
> With a neurological examination of a patient, **monosynaptic reflexes** are triggered by tapping the tendons of the Mm. biceps and triceps brachii with a rubber hammer. Thereby the spinal segments C5 and C6 are tested by tapping the tendon reflex of the biceps, and the spinal segments C6 and C7 are tested by tapping the tendon reflex of the triceps.

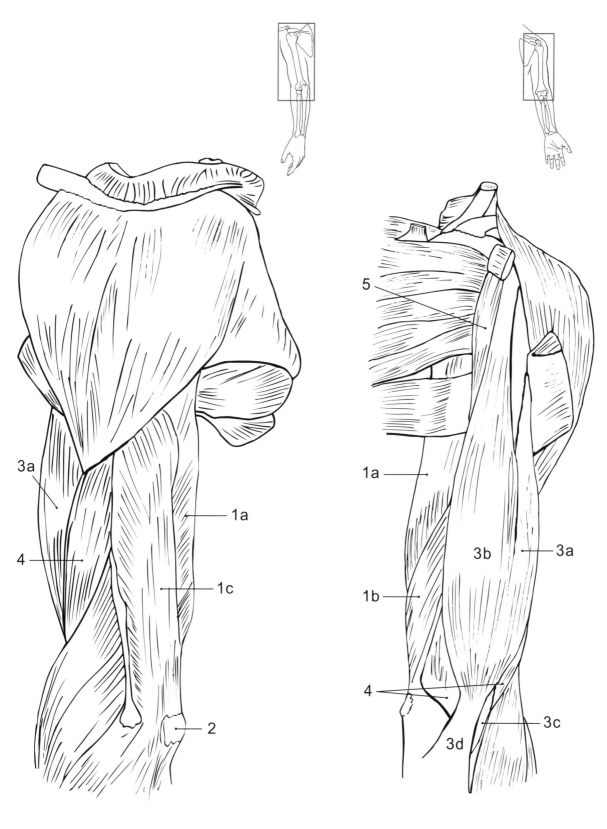

Abb. 2.3

2.4 Muscles of the forearm

The muscles of the forearm are divided into three groups:
- **radial muscles** (extensor)
- **dorsal muscles** (superficial and deep layer)
- **volar muscles** (superficial, intermediate and deep layer)

Only those muscles depicted in the figures are discussed.

Radial muscles The radial muscles originate furthest proximal to the humerus.

An example of these muscles is the **M. extensor carpi radialis longus (1)**. It originates from the side of the radial humerus and from the Septum intermusculare laterale and inserts at the Os metacarpale II.

The **M. extensor carpi radialis brevis (2)** originates from the Epicondylus lateralis humeri, runs along the M. extensor carpi radialis longus through the 2nd layer of tendons (➤ Chap. 2.6) and attaches onto the Os metacarpale III. Like the M. extensor carpi radialis longus dorsal, it extends the wrist joint.

M. brachioradialis also belongs to this group of muscles (not shown).

The innervation of the radial muscles is made via the N. radialis.

Dorsal muscles The dorsal muscles originate from the Epicondylus lateralis humeri.

An example of the superficial muscles of this group is the **M. extensor carpi ulnaris (3)**. It runs through the 6th layer of tendons and attaches at the Os metacarpale V.

The **M. supinator (4)** can be seen on the deep layer of these muscles. It originates at the dorsal surface of the **ulna (5)** and encompasses the proximal end of the **radius (6)** in a spiral pathway. Together with the M. biceps brachii, the M. supinator is the most important supinator of the forearm.

The dorsal muscles are innervated by the N. radialis.

Volar muscles The volar muscles are mostly found on the ulnar side of the forearm.

From the **superficial layer** one recognises the **M. pronator teres (7)**. It originates with two heads from the Epicondylus medialis humeri and from the Proc. coronoideus ulnae. The muscle then runs distally and radially and inserts distal of the M. supinator at the radius. The M. pronator teres is penetrated and also innervated by the N. medianus. It pronates the forearm and flexes in the elbow joint.

A further (visible) muscle of the superficial layer is the **M. palmaris longus (8)**, which originates from the Epicondylus me-

dialis humeri and runs as the only muscle of the volar muscles via the Retinaculum flexorum. The M. palmaris longus radiates into the **palmar aponeurosis (9)**. It flexes in the proximal wrist joint and elbow joint.

The **M. flexor carpi ulnaris (10)** also belongs to the superficial layer of the Epicondylus medialis and originates from the proximal third of the ulna and inserts via the **Os pisiforme (11)** as the sesamoid bone at the Ossa metacarpalia IV and V.

The **M. flexor carpi radialis (12)** originates from the Epicondylus medialis humeri and from the Fascia antebrachii, runs through the carpal tunnel and attaches at the Ossa metacarpalia II and III.

Note

The **volar muscles** are innervated by the **N. medianus**. The M. flexor carpi ulnaris and both the ulnar heads of the M. flexor digitorum profundus are exceptions as they are innervated by the N. ulnaris.

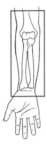
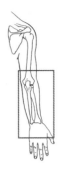

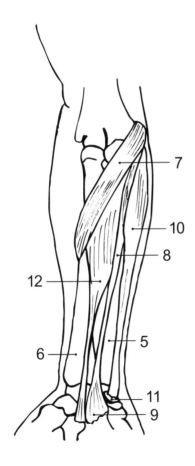
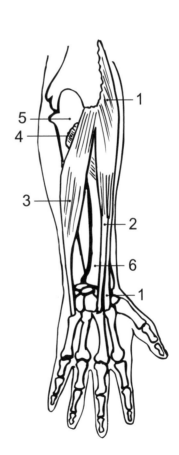

Abb. 2.4

2.5 Elbow joint (Articulatio cubiti)

Structure   The elbow joint is a compound joint with three parts. Here the distal part of the **humerus (1)** articulates with the proximal sections of the **radius (2)** and the **ulna (3).**

- In the **humeroulnar joint** the **Trochlea humeri (1a)** articulates with the **Incisura trochlearis (3a)** of the ulna. Thereby the ulnar 'forceps' of the **olecranon (3b)** grips from one side and the **Processus coronoideus (3c)** from the other side, as far around as the Trochlea humeri, so that this joint section has a distinctly bony formation and support. The humeroulnar joint is a **hinge joint**, in that the forearm can flex and extend.

- This movement also takes place in the **radioulnar joint**. Here the **Capitulum humeri (1b)** connects with the **Fovea articularis (2a)** of the **radial head (2b)**. Morphologically this is a **ball joint.** As the radius and ulna are securely connected via ligaments (Membrana interossea) with each other, it is also only a flexing and extending movement of the forearms that can take place here.

- The third partial joint of the Articulatio cubiti is located between the **Circumferentia articularis (2c)** of the radial head and the **Incisura radialis (3d)** of the ulna. The latter forms the small bony socket which is augmented by the **Ligamentum anulare radii (4)** to become a ring. This joint is a **rotary joint** and is described as a **proximal radio-ulnar joint**. Because the radius winds itself around the ulna, the hand can pronate or supinate in this joint (interacting with the distal radioulnar joint).

Ligaments   All joint surfaces of the three bones connected to the Articulatio cubiti, as well as the **Fossa coronoidea (1c)**, are encompassed by the **joint capsule (5)**. The elbow joint also has supporting ligament connections: the **Ligamentum collaterale ulnare (6)** runs from the **Epicondylus medialis (1d)** of the humerus to the ulna, and the **Ligamentum collaterale radiale (7)** runs from the **Epicondylus lateralis (1e)** of the humerus to the Ligamentum annulare radii.

In the picture on the right, the tendon of the **M. biceps brachii (8)** is visible, attached at the **Tuberositas radii (2d)**. The M. biceps brachii is an important supinator and enables the radius to move in the radioulnar joints.

Clinical remarks

Due to its strong bone conduction, elbow dislocations are rare. A sudden and violent pull on the forearm can however cause a dislocation of the radial head from the Ligamentum annulare radii (nursemaid's elbow).

More often, painful inflammations can appear around the elbow joint in the area where the forearm muscles attach to the medial and lateral Epicondylus humeri. These are often due to over-exertion during occupational or sport-related activities (e.g. tennis elbow).

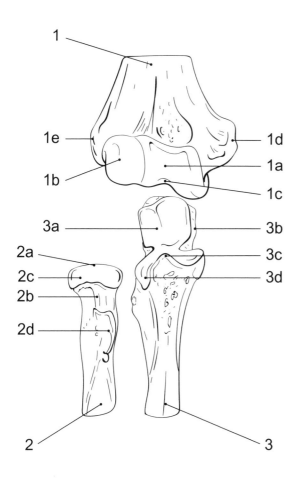

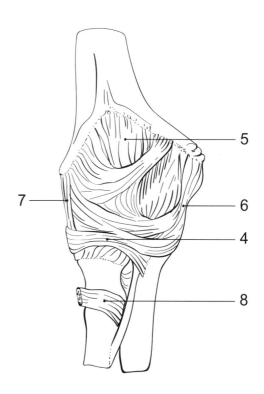

Abb. 2.5

2.6 Wrist joint (Articulatio manus)

The wrist joint (Art. manus) is divided into:
- the **proximal**
- the **distal** wrist joint

Proximal wrist joint (Art. radiocarpalis)   The **radius (1)** and the proximal row of carpal bones form the proximal wrist joint.
The proximal carpal bones are:
- **Os scaphoideum (scaphoid bone, 2)**
- **Os lunatum (lunate bone, 3)**
- **Os triquetrum (triquetral bone, 4)**
- **Os pisiforme (pisiform bone, 5)**

The first three bones mentioned form the common smooth, elliptical condyle, which join via a Discus articularis with the radius. The **Os pisiforme (pisiform bone, 5)**, instead of being part of the proximal wrist joint, is connected as a sesamoid bone in the attaching tendon of the M. flexor carpi ulnaris. The proximal wrist joint is a condyloid joint, because the hand is capable of dorsiflexion and palmar flexion, with ulnar or radial deviation.

Distal wrist joint (Art. mediocarpalis)   The distal wrist joint is between the proximal and the distal row of the carpal bones and the carpometacarpal joints are between the distal row of the carpal bones and the Ossa metacarpalia.
The distal row of the carpal bones constitute:
- the **Os trapezium (trapezium bone, 6)**
- the **Os trapezoideum (trapezoid bone, 7)**
- the **Os capitatum (capitate bone, 8)**
- the **Os hamatum (hamate bone, 9)**

Between the distal carpal bones and the Ossa metacarpalia II–IV there are very tight ligaments allowing only minimal movement. An exception is the flexible connection between the Os metacarpale V and the **Os hamatum (9),** which has more movement and facilitates the opposition of the little finger.
The **Os trapezium (6)** forms a saddle joint with the **Os metacarpale I (10)** in that the thumb can be opposed as well as abducted and adducted.

Note

The way in which the carpal bones are arranged can be remembered with the following mnemonics for the proximal and the distal rows:
Sam Likes To Push The Toy Car Hard. Straight Line To Pinky, Here Comes The Thumb.

Clinical remarks

Fractures of the carpal bones   If falling onto the hand in a radial and abducted position, the Os scaphoideum is often affected. Clinical signs are pain from an impacted fracture of the 2nd finger and pressure pain in the Foveola radialis. Because the Os scaphoideum is involved in almost all movements of the hand, a fracture requires a lengthy period in a cast.

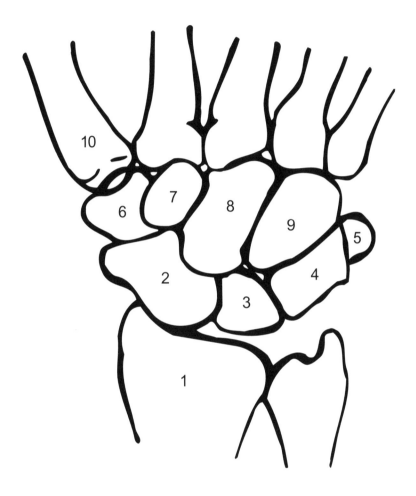

Abb. 2.6

2.7 Dorsal carpus and hand

On the dorsal side of the carpus, the Fascia antebrachii and the dorsal fascia of the hand connect with each other and become the strong, transversely running **Retinaculum extensorum (1)**. Underneath the Retinaculum extensorum, the dorsal and radial muscles of the forearm, enveloped by synovial tendon sheaths, run through six tendon compartments to the hand.

Tendon compartments
- **1st tendon compartment**
  The **M. abductor pollicis longus (2)** and the **M. extensor pollicis brevis (3)** run through the 1st tendon compartment. Both originate from the middle third of the ulna, from the Membrana interossea and from the radius. The M. abductor pollicis longus attaches at the base of the Os metacarpale I, and the M. extensor pollicis brevis at the proximal phalanx of the thumb. Both abduct the thumb and are innervated by the N. radialis.
- **2nd tendon compartment**
  The **M. extensor carpi radialis longus (4)** and the **M. extensor carpi radialis brevis (5)** run through the 2nd tendon compartment. The M. extensor carpi radialis longus originates from the radial side of the humerus and inserts at the Os metacarpale II. The M. extensor carpi radialis brevis originates from the Epicondylus lateralis and inserts at the Os metacarpale III. Both muscles are innervated by the N. radialis. They make a dorsal flexion of the hand possible. Additionally, the M. extensor carpi radialis longus makes radial abduction in the wrist joint possible.
- **3rd tendon compartment**
  The **M. extensor pollicis longus (6)** runs through the 3rd tendon compartment. It comes from the middle third of the ulna and from the Membrana interossea and attaches at the distal phalanx of the thumb. It is innervated by the N. radialis. The M. extensor pollicis longus elongates the proximal and distal phalanx and adducts the thumb.
- **4th tendon compartment**
  The **M. extensor digitorum (7)** and the **M. extensor indicis (8)** run through the 4th tendon compartment. The **M. extensor digitorum** originates from the Epicondylus lateralis humeri and radiates into the **dorsal aponeurosis (9)** of the IInd–Vth finger. The **M. extensor indicis** originates from the ulna and radiates into the dorsal aponeurosis of the index finger. Both muscles extend in the wrist joint and in the finger joints of the corresponding finger. They are innervated by N. radialis.

- **5th tendon compartment**
  The **M. extensor digiti minimi (10)** runs through the 5th tendon compartment. It originates via a tendon from the Epicondylus lateralis, radiates into the dorsal aponeurosis of the little finger and extends into its joints. It is innervated by the N. radialis.
- **6th tendon compartment**
  The **M. extensor carpi ulnaris (11)** runs through the 6th tendon compartment. It originates from the Epicondylus lateralis and from the dorsal side of the ulna and inserts at the Os metacarpale V. The M. extensor carpi ulnaris enables ulnar abduction and dorsal flexion (extension) in the wrist joint. It is also innervated by the N. radialis.

Mm. interossei dorsales Four **Mm. interossei dorsales (12)** are stretched across the Ossa metacarpalia. They enable spreading of the fingers, flexing at the metacarpophalangeal joint and extending at the interphalangeal joint. The Mm. interossei dorsales are innervated by the N. ulnaris.

Note

Tendon compartment	Muscle
1.	M. abductor pollicis longus, M. extensor pollicis brevis
2.	M. extensor carpi radialis longus, M. extensor carpi radialis brevis
3.	M. extensor pollicis longus
4.	M. extensor digitorum, M. extensor indicis
5.	M. extensor digiti minimi
6.	M. extensor carpi ulnari

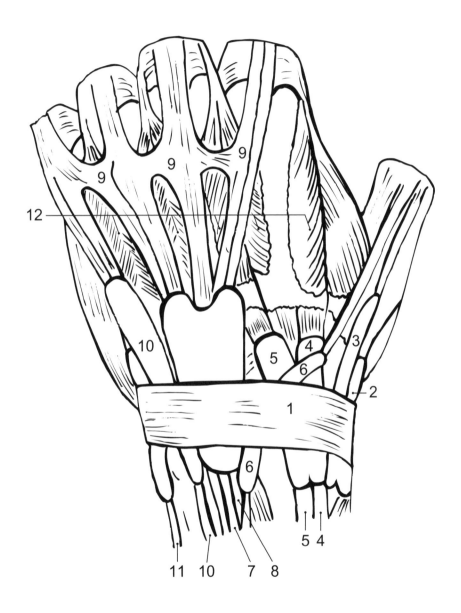

Abb. 2.7

2.8 Volar side of the distal forearm and the hand

The volar group of forearm muscles consist of:
- the **superficial layer** with the M. pronator teres, M. flexor carpi radialis, M. palmaris longus, M. flexor carpi ulnaris (➤ Chap. 2.4)
- the **intermediate layer** with the M. flexor digitorum superficialis
- the **deep layer** with the M. flexor digitorum profundus, M. flexor pollicis longus, M. pronator quadratus

M. pronator quadratus The **M. pronator quadratus (1)** is located on the Membrana interossea on the volar side of the distal forearm. It runs from the **ulna (2)** to the **radius (3)** and pronates the forearm. The M. pronator quadratus is innervated by the N. interosseus from the N. medianus.

Carpal tunnel The Canalis carpi (carpal tunnel) is located between the carpal bones and the **Retinaculum flexorum (4,** opened here). It serves as a passageway to the hand for the tendons of the forearm flexors:
- The **M. flexor carpi radialis (5)** runs furthest radially through the carpal tunnel. It comes from the Epicondylus medialis and from the fascia of the forearm and inserts at the base of the Os metacarpale II. The M. flexor carpi radialis induces a palmar flexion in the wrist joint and is innervated by the N. medianus.
- The **M. flexor pollicis longus (6)** originates from the palmar surface of the radius and the Membrana interossea and runs to the distal phalanx of the thumb. Most importantly it is used to flex the thumb and helps it to be oppositional. It is innervated by the N. medianus.
- In the centre of the carpal tunnel, one can see the four tendons of the **M. flexor digitorum profundus (7)**. The M. flexor digitorum profundus originates from the front of the ulna, the Membrana interossea and the fascia of the forearm and attaches at the end of the phalanges of the fingers II–V. Thereby its tendons penetrate the bifurcated tendons of the **M. flexor digitorum superficialis (8)**, which insert at the middle phalanges. The rest of its tendons and the M. flexor digitorum superficialis itself have been removed in the illustration. The M. flexor digitorum profundus flexes all the hand and finger joints II–V. Both its radial heads are innervated by the N. medianus, the ulnar heads of the N. ulnaris.
- The **M. flexor digitorum superficialis (8)** originates from the Epicondylus medialis and from the Proc. coronoideus ulnae, and runs more superficially than the M. flexor digito-

rum profundus on the forearm. The M. flexor digitorum superficialis is innervated by the N. medianus. The M. flexor digitorum superficialis flexes in the wrist joint and in the middle and metacarpophalangeal joints of the fingers II–V.
- The **M. flexor carpi ulnaris (9)** originates from the Epicondylus medialis humeri and from the ulna. It uses the **Os pisiforme (10)** as a sesamoid bone and then attaches to the base of the Os metacarpale V. It is innervated by the N. ulnaris.

Muscles of the thenar eminence (thenar muscles) The **M. abductor pollicis brevis (11)**, the superficial head of the **M. flexor pollicis brevis (12)** and the **M. opponens pollicis (13)** originate from the Retinaculum flexorum. They insert at the sesamoid bone in the capsule of the thumb basal joint and at the radial sides of the Os metacarpale I. They abduct and/or oppose the thumb, or flex in the metacarpophalangeal joint. These muscles are innervated by the N. medianus. The Caput profundum of the M. flexor pollicis brevis originates from the Os trapezium and Os capitatum. The **M. adductor pollicis (14)** emerges with its Caput obliquum from the bases of the Ossa metacarpalia II–IV, and with its Caput transversum from the palmar side of the Os metacarpale III. The M. adductor pollicis and the Caput profundum of the M. flexor pollicis brevis are innervated by the R. profundus of the N. ulnaris.

Muscles of the hypothenar eminence (hypothenar muscles) The hypothenar eminence is composed of the **M. flexor digiti minimi (15)**, **M. opponens digiti minimi (16)** and the **M. abductor digiti minimi (17)**. They originate from the Retinaculum flexorum and/or from the Os pisiforme and are innervated by the N. ulnaris.

Muscles of the palm of the hand The muscles of the palm of the hand are composed of the:
- **Mm. lumbricales (18)**
- **Mm. interossei dorsales** (➤ Chap. 2.7)
- **Mm. interossei palmares** (➤ Chap. 2.9)

The **Mm. lumbricales (18)** originate from the tendons of the M. flexor digitorum profundus and radiate into the dorsal aponeuroses of the fingers II–V. They extend the terminal tendons and flex the interphalangeal and the metacarpophalangeal joints. Both radial Mm. lumbricales are innervated by the N. medianus, and the lumbar Mm. lumbricales by the N. ulnaris.

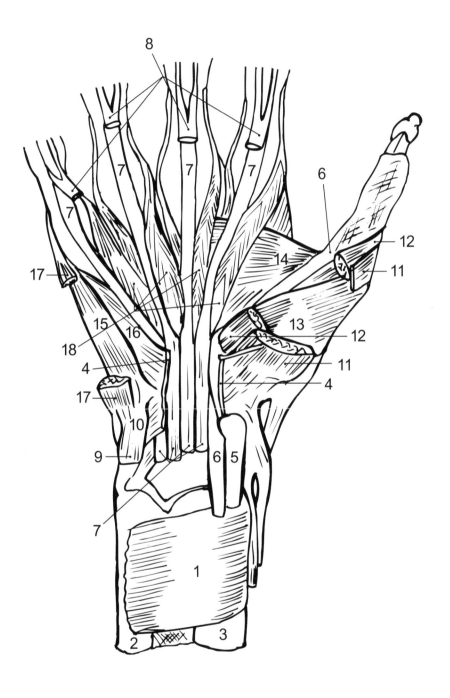

Abb. 2.8

2.9 Short muscles of the hand

The muscles of the hand which are attached to and originate in the area of the hand are divided into:

- muscles of the thenar eminence
- muscles of the palm of the hand
- muscles of the hypothenar eminence

Muscles of the thenar eminence (Thenar muscles, ➤ Chap. 2.8) The **M. opponens pollicis (2)** is visible after removing the **M. abductor pollicis brevis (1)**. The **Caput profundum** of the **M. flexor pollicis brevis (3)**, as well as the **Caput transversum (4a)** and the **Caput obliquum (4b)** of the **M. adductor pollicis** have been severed.

Muscles of the palm of the hand The three **Mm. interossei palmares (5)** originate from the ulnar side of the Os metacarpale II and from the radial side of the Ossa metacarpalia III and IV. They insert at the proximal phalanx and the dorsal aponeuroses of the fingers II, IV and V. They flex at the metacarpophalangeal joints and extend at the interphalangeal joints. They also adduct the fingers by moving them towards the middle finger.

The **Mm. lumbricales (6)** originate from the tendons of the M. flexor digitorum profundus and radiate into the dorsal aponeuroses of the fingers II–V. They extend the terminal tendons and flex the interphalangeal and metacarpophalangeal joints. Both the radial Mm. lumbricales are innervated by the N. medianus, and both the ulnar Mm. lumbricales by the N. ulnaris.

Muscles of the hypothenar eminence (Hypothenar muscles, ➤ Chap. 2.8) After severing the **M. abductor digiti minimi (7)**, the **M. flexor digiti minimi brevis (8)** and the **M. opponens digiti minimi (9)** become visible.

Clinical remarks

Injury to the N. ulnaris is the second most common peripheral nerve lesion. It can be triggered by trauma or through chronic pressure injury (e.g. in the Sulcus nervi ulnaris on the olecranon). Besides sensory disturbance in the hand (➤ Chap. 2.12), disorders of the Mm. interossei and the hypothenar musculature can occur, presenting as **claw hand**.

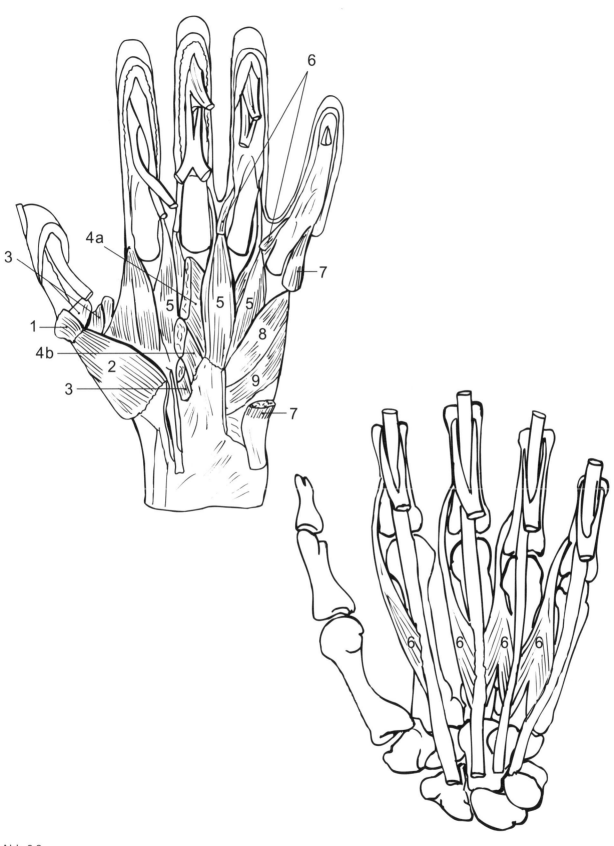

Abb. 2.9

2.10 Plexus brachialis

The Plexus brachialis is formed by the Rr. anteriores of the spinal nerves C5–Th1. The vertebrae are marked as CV-ThI in the illustration to help with orientation. The following are found at the lateral margin of the M. scalenus anterior:

- the Rr. anteriores from the C5 and C6 to the **Truncus superior (1)**
- the R. anterior from the C7 to the **Truncus medius (2)**
- the Rr. anteriores from the C8 and the Th1 to the **Truncus inferior (3)**

The nerves of the supraclavicular part of the Plexus brachialis (Pars supraclavicularis) descend as early as above the clavicula. The **three fascicles** of the Plexus brachialis emerge from the trunci below the clavicula: the three trunci each divide into a ventral and a dorsal branch. The dorsal branches combine to form the **Fasciculus posterior (4)**. The ventral branches of the upper and middle trunk combine to form the **Fasciculus lateralis (5)**, and the ventral branch of the Truncus inferior forms the **Fasciculus medialis (6)**. The three fascicles lie dorsally, laterally and/or medially of the A. axillaris (➤ Chap. 2.11).

Fasciculus posterior The Fasciculus posterior provides the **N. axillaris (7)**, which runs into the lateral axilla and innervates the M. deltoideus and the M. teres minor. The **N. radialis (8)** also exits from the Fasciculus posterior. It gyrates around the humerus in the Sulcus nervi radialis, innervates the M. triceps brachii and reaches the elbow. There it divides into an R. profundus and an R. superficialis. The R. profundus penetrates the M. supinator and innervates the dorsal and radial groups of the forearm muscles. The R. superficialis runs parallel to the M. brachioradialis on the surface and sensorily innervates half of the dorsal side of the hand and the radial 2½ of the finger.

Fasciculus lateralis The **N. musculocutaneus (9)** emerges from the Fasciculus lateralis, penetrating the M. coracobrachialis and innervating the flexors on the forearm. The Fasciculus lateralis also provides the **Radix lateralis (10a)** of the **N. medianus (10)**.

Fasciculus medialis Its **Radix medialis (10b)**, along with the Radix lateralis from the Fasciculus lateralis, forms the **median fork (10c)** around the A. axillaris. The **N. medianus (10)** runs in the Sulcus bicipitalis medialis to the elbow, penetrates through both the heads of the M. pronator teres and runs between the superficial and deep flexors of the forearms to the carpal tunnel. It innervates most of the flexors and the prona-

tors on the forearm. After passing through the carpal tunnel it divides into branches for the muscles for the thenar eminence and the radial Mm. lumbricales, as well as into cutaneous branches for the radial 3½ finger on the palmar side.

The **N. ulnaris (11)** also exits from the Fasciculus medialis. It runs in the Sulcus bicipitalis medialis to the olecranon, through the Sulcus nervi ulnaris and parallel along the forearm to the M. flexor carpi ulnaris. There it innervates both the ulnar heads of the M. flexor digitorum profundus and the M. flexor carpi ulnaris. At the wrist joint it divides into an R. profundus and an R. superficialis. Both run via the Retinaculum flexorum. The **R. superficialis** sensorily innervates the 1½ ulnar fingers on the palmar side and the 2½ ulnar fingers on the dorsal side of the hand. The **R. profundus** innervates the muscles of the hypothenar eminence as well as of the thenar eminence of the M. adductor pollicis and the Caput profundum of the M. flexor pollicis brevis.

The **N. cutaneus brachii medialis (12)** and the **N. cutaneus antebrachii medialis (13)** are further branches of the Fasciculus medialis.

Clinical remarks

Proximal **lesions of the N. radialis** (e.g. with a fracture of the humeral shaft) result in **wrist drop,** which is caused by the failure of the extensors on the forearm.

Through proximal **damage to the N. medianus,** the majority of the flexors, amongst others, fail on the forearm. When asked to make a fist, the patient can only make an **oath hand,** as the 4th and 5th fingers can still be flexed, using the heads of the M. flexor digitorum profundus, innervated by the N. ulnaris.

Injuries to the N. ulnaris, with failure of the Mm. interossei, lead to **claw hand.**

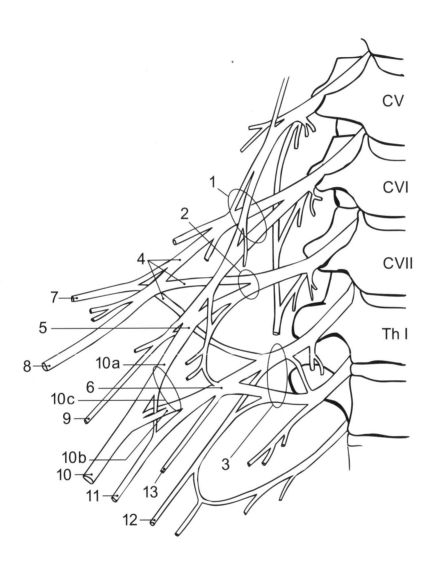

CV

CVI

CVII

Th I

Abb. 2.10

2.11 Nerves of the forearm

In the axilla, one can see the fascicles of the Plexus brachialis around the **A. axillaris (1)**:
- dorsally, the **Fasciculus posterior (2)**
- medially, the **Fasciculus medialis (3)**
- laterally, the **Fasciculus lateralis (4)**

Fasciculus posterior   The **N. axillaris (5)** emerges from the Fasciculus posterior. It runs from the axilla in the lateral axillary gap and innervates the M. deltoideus and the M. teres minor. As a further branch of the Fasciculus posterior, the **N. radialis (6)** runs to the humerus. Here it disappears along with the **A. profunda brachii (7)** into the depths and gyrates through the Sulcus nervi radialis around the dorsal side of the humerus, where it innervates the M. triceps brachii.

Fasciculus lateralis   The **N. musculocutaneus (8)** emerges from the Fasciculus lateralis. It penetrates the **M. coracobrachialis (9)** and innervates it as well as the **M. brachialis (10)** and the **M. biceps brachii (11)**. The lateral root of the **N. medianus (12)** emerges from the Fasciculus lateralis.

Fasciculus medialis   The second root of the N. medianus emerges from the Fasciculus medialis, so that the **median fork (12a)** is formed around the A. axillaris. The N. medianus passes in the Sulcus bicipitalis medialis on the forearm, along with the **A. brachialis (13)** and the **N. ulnaris (14)**, a further branch from the Fasciculus medialis. The N. ulnaris then runs to the olecranon and there runs in the Sulcus nervi ulnaris.

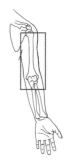

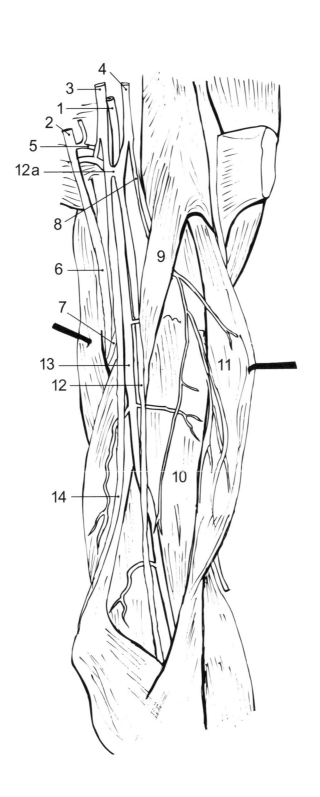

Abb. 2.11

2.12 Pathways of the hand

Blood Vessels   On the distal forearm one can feel the pulse of the **A. radialis (1)** next to the tendon of the **M. flexor carpi radialis (2)**. Further distally, the A. radialis turns to dorsal and ends up in the snuff box (not shown). The **A. ulnaris (3)** lies on the distal forearm next to the tendon of the **M. flexor carpi ulnaris (4)**.

The vessels of the hand and fingers are supplied from the **Arcus palmaris superficialis (superficial palmar arch, 5)** and the **Arcus palmaris profundus** (not shown).

The **Arcus palmaris superficialis (5)** is fed by a strong inflow from the A. ulnaris, which runs via the **Retinaculum flexorum (6)** along the carpus and then in an arch over the palm of the hand. The **A. radialis (1)** provides only a small **R. palmaris superficialis (1a)** to the superficial palmar arch.

With the **Arcus palmaris profundus (deep palmar arch**, not shown), the opposite is the case. The **A. ulnaris (3)** provides a small **R. palmaris profundus (3a)**, which anastomoses on the bases of the Ossa metacarpalia II–IV with a large inflow from the A. radialis. From the Arcus palmaris superficialis, the **Aa. digitales palmares communes (7)** exit to the metacarpophalangeal joints. There they divide into the **Aa. digitales palmares propriae (8)**.

Nerves   The **N. medianus (9)** runs between the tendons of the **superficial** and the **deep finger benders (10)** below the **Retinaculum flexorum (6)** through the carpal tunnel. On the hand it provides short branches to the thenar eminence musculature and branches off into the **Nn. digitales palmares communes (11)** for the radial 3½ fingers. In the area of the metacarpophalangeal joints, these divide into the **Nn. digitales palmares proprii (12)**, which run along the radial and ulnar margins of the fingers.

The **N. ulnaris (13)** lies on the distal forearm next to the A. ulnaris. It runs via the Retinaculum flexorum and divides into the **R. superficialis (13a)** and a **R. profundus (13b)**. The R. superficialis provides the Nn. digitales palmares communes to the 1½ ulnar fingers. The R. profundus penetrates the hypothenar eminence musculature and innervates this as well as parts of the thenar eminence musculature (➤ Chap. 2.8).

Note

Sensory innervation of the hand

- N. medianus
- N. radialis
- N. ulnaris

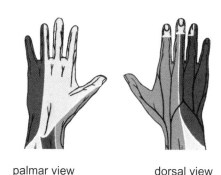

palmar view   dorsal view

Abb. 2.12 View from palmar – View from dorsal

Clinical remarks

Median nerve palsy is the most common peripheral nerve lesion. The N. medianus can be compromised, especially in older women, in the area of the carpal tunnel through inflammation, trauma or idiopathically **(carpal tunnel syndrome)**. Symptoms manifest especially at night as pain felt in the hand, and later on also as sensory disturbances in the innervation area of the N. medianus, as well as failure and eventually atrophy of the thenar eminence musculature.

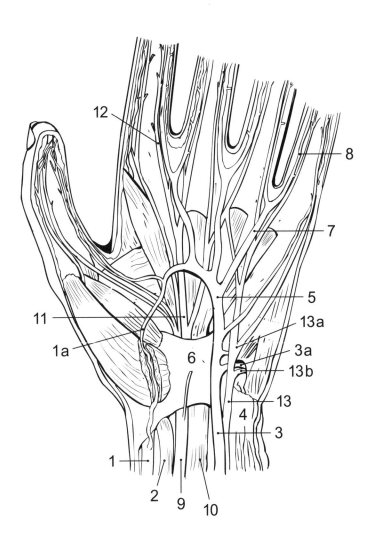

Abb. 2.13

2.13 Cross-sections through the upper and forearm

Cross-section through the mid-upper arm On the cross-section through the upper arm, the **humerus (1)** and the **Septa intermuscularia brachii mediale (2)** and **laterale (3)** are visible, separating the extensor compartment from the flexor compartment of the upper arm.

In the **flexor compartment,** the **M. biceps brachii (4)** is visible and on the humerus the **M. brachialis (5)**. Between the muscles, a section of the **N. musculocutaneus (6)** innervates the flexor on the upper arm.

In the **extensor compartment,** the **M. triceps brachii (7)** is visible with its three heads: the **Caput laterale (7a)**, **Caput mediale (7b)** and **Caput longum (7c)**. This muscle is innervated by the **N. radialis (8)**, which passes here in the Sulcus nervi radialis along with the **A. profunda brachii (9)** along the shaft of the humerus.

A neurovascular pathway containing the **A. brachialis (10)** and **V. brachialis (11)**, the **N. medianus (12)**, the **N. ulnaris (13)** and the **N. cutaneus antebrachii medialis (14)** runs in the Sulcus bicipitalis medialis.

Cross-section through the mid-forearm On the cross-section one can see the **radius (15)** and the **ulna (16)**, which are connected with each other via the **Membrana interossea antebrachii (17)**.

Dorsal of the Membrana interossea, one can see sections of the muscles of the **dorsal group**:

- **M. extensor pollicis longus (18)**
- **M. extensor carpi ulnaris (19)**
- **M. extensor pollicis brevis (20)**
- **M. extensor digitorum (21)**

The **N. interosseus antebrachii posterior (22)** passes from the N. radialis and the **A. and V. interossea posterior (23)** between the muscles.

Around the radius are the muscles of the **radial group**:

- **M. extensor carpi radialis brevis (24)**
- **M. extensor carpi radialis longus (25)**
- **M. brachioradialis (26)**

One can also see the insertion point of the **M. pronator teres (27)** on the radius. Next to the M. brachioradialis are the **R. superficialis nervi radialis (8a)** and the **A. radialis (28)**.

Ventral of the Membrana interossea are the forearm flexors:

- **M. flexor digitorum profundus (29)**

- **M. flexor pollicis longus (30)**
- **M. flexor digitorum superficialis (31)**
- **M. flexor carpi radialis (32)**
- **M. palmaris longus (33)**
- **M. flexor carpi ulnaris (34)**

The **N. medianus (12)** passes between the superficial and deep finger flexors on the Membrana interossea of the **N. interosseus antebrachii anterior (35)** from the N. medianus along with the A. and V. interossea anterior. The **A. und V. ulnaris (36)** and the **N. ulnaris (13)** run parallel to the M. flexor carpi ulnaris.

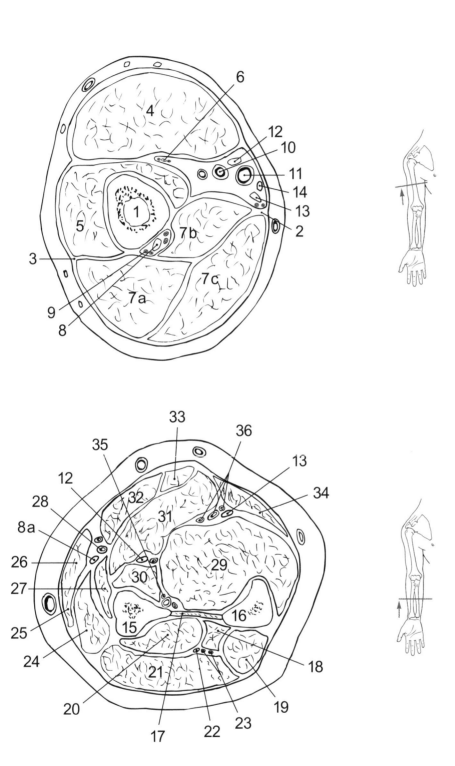

Abb. 2.14 f002-025-028-9780702052781

33

3.1 Pelvis

The bony pelvis (Os coxae) is shaped by:
- the **Os ilium (iliac bone, 1a–g)**
- the **Os ischii (seat bone, 2a–f)**
- the **Os pubis (pubic bone, 3a–c)**

The three bones meet in the socket of the hip joint, in the **acetabulum (4a–c)**.

Os ilium   The Os ilium (iliac bone) consists of a **corpus (1a)** and an **ala (1b)**. The Ala ossis ilii (ala of ilium) runs cranially in a bony protrusion, the **Crista iliaca (iliac crest, 1c)**. The Crista iliaca terminates ventrally in the **Spina iliaca anterior superior (1d)**. The **Spina iliaca anterior inferior (1e)** lies somewhat caudally. Dorsally, the Crista iliaca terminates in the **Spina iliaca posterior superior (1f)**, with the **Spina iliaca posterior inferior (1g)** lying somewhat caudally thereof.

Os ischii   At the Os ischii (seat bone) the **Corpus ossis ischii (2a)** can be seen as well as an archshaped part running into the **Tuber ischiadicum (ischial tuberosity, 2b)**. Dorsally, the arch extends up to the **Spina ischiadica (2c)**. Cranially of the Spina ischiadica there is a recess, the **Incisura ischiadica major (2d)**, and caudally, the **Incisura ischiadica minor (2e)**.

Os pubis   The most important bone structure of the Os pubis (pubic bone) is the **Corpus ossis pubis (3a)**. From the **Corpus ossis pubis (3a),** the **Ramus superior (3b)** runs to the Symphysis pubica. The **Ramus inferior (3c)** meets the **Ramus ossis ischii (2f)**, bordering the **Foramen obturatum (5)**. The Ossa pubis are connected through the symphysis.

Acetabulum   The acetabulum (socket of the hip joint) presents a **Facies lunata (4a)**, which articulates with the head of the femur. It is surrounded by a bony crest, the **Limbus acetabuli (4b)**. On the lower margin this is interrupted by the **Incisura acetabuli (4c)**.

Compounds of both the Os coxae   The bony pelvis develops from the two **Os coxae (6a und b)** merging with each other:
- ventrally through the **Symphysis pubica** (not shown)
- dorsally through the articulation with the **Os sacrum (7)** in the **iliosacral joint (8)**

The **iliosacral joint** is an amphiarthrosis (type of continuous slightly movable joint), making oscillating movements possible.

From the Os sacrum, the **Lig. sacrotuberale (9)** runs to the **Tuber ischiadicum (2b)** and the **Lig. sacrospinale (10)** runs to the **Spina ischiadica (2c)**. Thereby the **Incisura ischiadica major (2d)** to the Foramen ischiadicum majus and the **Incisura ischiadica minor (2e)** to the Foramen ischiadicum minus are bounded.

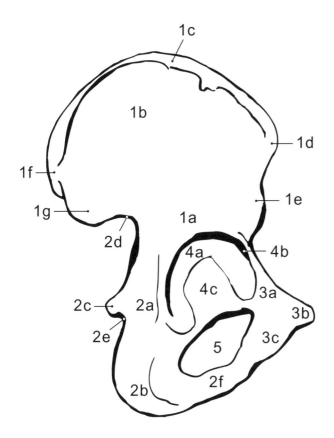

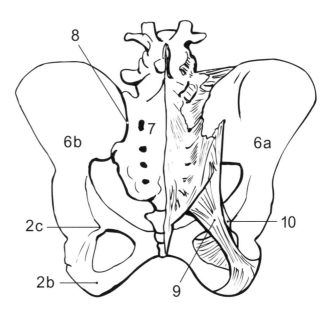

Abb. 3.1

3.2 Hip joint (Articulatio coxae)

Structure The hip joint consists of the bony pelvis (Os coxae) and the femur. The socket, the **acetabulum** (➤ Chap. 3.1), consists collectively of the **Os ilium (1),** the **Os ischii (2)** and the **Os pubis (3)**. When standing, the main burden is transferred to the Facies lunata of the acetabulum, which is partially covered with cartilage. The bony socket of the acetabulum is augmented with connective tissue, the Limbus acetabuli. This runs in a circle around the rim of the acetabulum and stretches over the equator of the joint head. Thereby a special type of ball joint is created, the so-called **cotyloid joint**. In the hip joint, the upper leg can be bent and straightened, abducted and adducted, as well as rotated inwards and outwards.

The joint head constitutes the **Caput femoris (4).** From here the **Ligamentum capitis femoris (5)** runs inside the joint capsule to the acetabulum. This ligament has no mechanical function, but contains the artery which is particularly important during development for the blood supply of the femoral head. The hip joint is enveloped by a strong joint capsule, strengthened with ligaments, which also encloses the **Collum femoris (6)**.

Ligaments The **Ligamentum illiofemorale (8)** runs ventrally in a fan-like shape to the **Trochanter minor (9)** of the femur under the **Spina iliaca anterior inferior (7)** of the Os ilii. It is the strongest ligament of the human body and inhibits extension and outwards rotation with its many different parts.

The **Ligamentum ischiofemorale (10)** radiates dorsally outwards from the **Corpus ossis ischii (11)** into the joint capsule in the area of the base of the **Trochanter major (12)** and **minor (9)**. It inhibits extreme adduction and inwards rotation.

The **Ligamentum pubofemorale (13)** ultimately runs ventrally of the parts of the Os pubis which adjoin the acetabulum to the base of the Trochanter minor and inhibits extreme abduction.

Clinical remarks

Hip joint dysplasia is a congenital malalignment of the hip joint, e.g. due to a hip joint socket that is too small. Treatment is mostly conservative, e.g. by swaddling the legs widely apart or with abduction pants. Without suitable treatment, hip join arthrosis can occur later in life.

The angle between the neck of the femur and the shaft of the femur normally amounts to approx. 127°. If it is less than 120°, it is called a **Coxa vara**, and if over 140° it is called a **Coxa valga**. These malalignments can be congenital (hip joint dysplasia) or acquired (e.g. rickets). The resulting chronic imbalance can cause premature arthrosis in the hip joint.

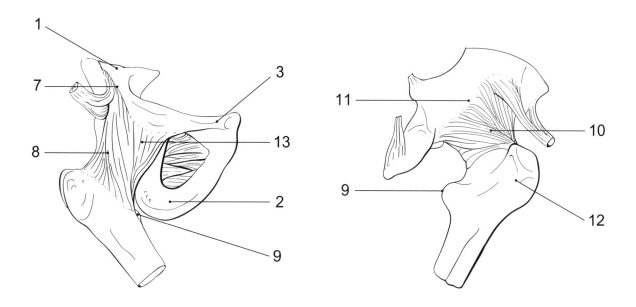

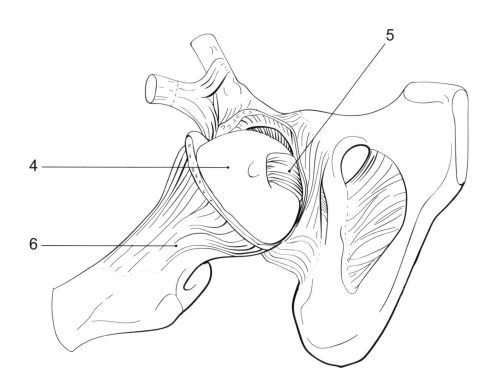

Abb. 3.2

3.3 Muscles of the gluteal region and hamstring muscles

Gluteal muscles   The following belong to the gluteal muscle group:

- **M. gluteus maximus (1)**
- **M. gluteus medius (2)**
- **M. gluteus minimus (3)**

The **M. gluteus maximus (1)** originates from the Os sacrum, the Lig. sacrotuberale, the Crista iliaca and the Fascia thoracolumbalis. It ascends obliquely to lateral, attaches at the Tuberositas glutea of the femur and radiates into the Fascia lata and the Tractus iliotibialis. The M. gluteus maximus is the strongest extensor in the hip joint and rotates outwards. Its cranial fibres abduct and its caudal fibres adduct in the hip joint. It is innervated by the N. gluteus inferior.

The **M. gluteus medius (2)** originates in a fan shape from the outside of the Ala ossis ilii and inserts at the tip of the Trochanter major.

The **M. gluteus minimus (3)** is hidden by the M. gluteus medius on the outside of the Ala ossis ilii (= origin) and also runs up to the Trochanter major.

Both muscles are innervated by the N. gluteus superior. They abduct in the hip joint, and the ventral fibres induce an inwards rotation and the dorsal fibres an outwards rotation. When standing on one leg and when walking, the respectively contralateral Mm. glutei medius and minimus prevent the hip from dropping down on the side of the free leg.

Pelvitrochanteric muscles   This group of muscles consists of:

- **M. piriformis (4)**
- **M. obturatorius internus (5)**
- **M. obturatorius externus** (not shown)
- **Mm. gemelli superior (6) and inferior (7)**
- **M. quadratus femoris (8)**

The six small muscles of this group originate from the Os sacrum or the Os ischii and run almost horizontally to the Trochanter major.

The **M. piriformis (4)** comes from the ventral side of the Os sacrum from the lesser pelvis and leaves it via the Foramen ischiadicum majus. Thereby it divides it into the **Foramina supra- (9)** and the **infrapiriforme (10)**. It induces an outwards rotation and abducts in the hip joint.

The **M. obturatorius internus (5)** originates in the inner pelvis at the Foramen obturatum, uses the Incisura ischiadica minor as a deflection guide (hypomochlion) and inserts at the Trochanter major.

The **Mm. gemelli superior (6)** and **inferior (7)** lie on both sides of the M. obturatorius internus. They originate from the Spina ischiadica and/or from the Tuber ischiadicum. Both the muscles work as outward rotators.

The **M. quadratus femoris (8)** runs from the Tuber ischiadicum to the Crista intertrochanterica. It induces outward rotation and adduction.

> **Note**
>
> **Innervation of the pelvitrochanteric muscles**
> M. piriformis → N. ischiadus and/or N. musculi piriformis (Plexus sacralis)
> M. obturatorius internus, Mm. gemelli superior and inferior → N. musculi obturatorii interni and Rr. musculares (Plexus sacralis) (Plexus sacralis)
> M. quadratus femoris → N. musculi quadrati femoris (Plexus sacralis)

Hamstring muscles   The hamstring muscles are both extensors in the hip joint as well as flexors in the knee joint. The following belong to this group:

- **M. biceps femoris (11)** with the Caput longum and the Caput breve
- **M. semitendinosus (12**
- **M. semimembranosus (13)**.

This muscle group originates from the Tuber ischiadicum and runs to the lower leg.

The **M. biceps femoris (11)** originates additionally with its Caput breve from the Linea aspera of the femur. It inserts at the Caput fibulae and can thereby also enable the knee joint to rotate outwards.

The **M. semitendinosus (12)** inserts via the Pes anserinus superficialis at the Tuberositas tibiae. With this process it enables the knee joint to rotate inwards.

The attaching tendon of the **M. semimembranosus (13)** constitutes the Pes anserinus profundus on the Epicondylus medialis tibiae and enables the knee joint to rotate inwards.

Note

Innervation of the hamstring muscles
All hamstring muscles → N. tibialis
Exception: M. biceps femoris, Caput breve → N. fibularis

Clinical remarks

With a **disorder of the Mm. glutei medius and minimus,** the pelvis tilts when walking to the side of the free leg and that causes a waddling gait, accompanied by a side-to-side movement of the trunk (Trendelenburg gait).

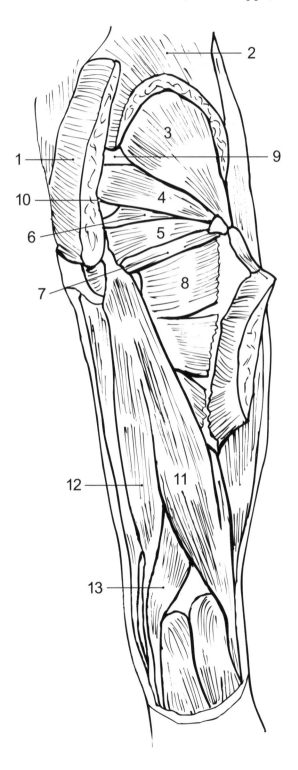

Abb. 3.3

39

3.4 Ventral muscles of the upper leg

Seen from the ventral side of the upper leg one can differentiate two muscle groups:

- extensors
- adductors

Extensors   The **M. quadriceps femoris (1a–e)** consists of four heads:

- **M. rectus femoris (1a)**
- **M. vastus intermedius (1b)**
- **M. vastus lateralis (1c)**
- **M. vastus medialis (1d)**

These unite to become a common terminal tendon, the **Lig. patellae (1e)**, and attach at the Tuberositas tibiae. In the Lig. patellae, the **Patella (2)** is engaged as a sesamoid bone. The M. quadriceps femoris is the only extensor in the knee joint.

The **M. rectus femoris (1a)** originates from the Spina iliaca anterior inferior and is thereby the only one of the four heads with two joints. It also flexes the hip joint.

The **M. vastus intermedius (1b)** originates from the front of the femur and lies underneath the M. rectus femoris.

Both of the **Mm. vastus lateralis (1c)** and **vastus medialis (1d)** originate from the dorsally situated Linea aspera and cover the femur laterally and/or medially.

The **M. sartorius (3)** has been extensively removed here. It originates from the Spina iliaca anterior superior, and its terminal tendon forms the Pes anserinus superficialis in conjunction with the M. semitendinosus (➢ Chap. 3.3) and the M. gracilis at the medial knee joint margin. It rotates inwards in the knee joint, outwards in the hip joint and flexes in both joints.

Adductors   From the ventral side, some of the adductors can be seen.

The **M. gracilis (4)** originates as a slim muscle from the Ramus inferior ossis pubis. Besides its function as an adductor, it can flex the hip and knee joint as well as rotate inwards in the knee joint. Its terminal tendon helps to form the Pes anserinus superficialis.

The **M. adductor brevis (5)** originates from the Ramus inferior ossis pubis and runs to the proximal third of the Linea aspera.

The **M. pectineus (6)** originates laterally from it, from the Pecten ossis pubis. It inserts caudally of the Trochanter minor at the Linea pectinea.

The **M. adductor magnus (7)** originates from the Ramus inferior ossis pubis up to the Tuber ischiadicum. It inserts at the Linea aspera and down to the Tuberculum adductorium at the Epicondylus medialis of the femur.

The **M. adductor longus (8)** has been severed in the illustration. It originates at the Os pubis and runs to the middle third of the Linea aspera.

Besides their adduction functions, the Mm. adductores brevis and longus can flex and rotate outwards in the hip joint. The M. adductor magnus can also rotate outwards in the hip joint and can flex and stretch with its various parts.

Note

Innervation
Extensors, M. sartorius → N. femoralis
Adductors → N. obturatorius

Clinical remarks

The **proprioceptive reflex** can be tested by striking the patellar tendon with a percussion hammer, thereby testing the spinal cord segments L3–4.

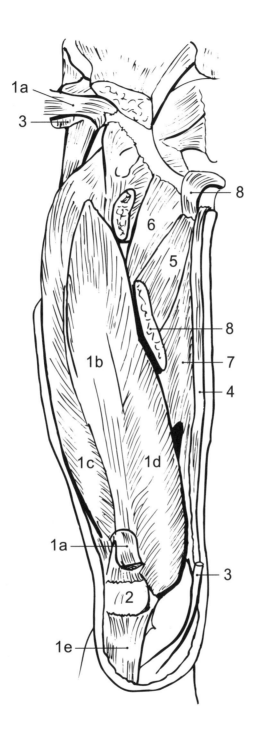

1a

3

8

6

5

8

1b

7

4

1c

1d

1a

3

2

1e

Abb. 3.4

3.5 Knee joint (Articulatio genus)

The knee joint (Art. genus) is a compound joint, in which the **femoral condyles (1a and b)** articulate with the **tibial condyles (2a and b)** and the **patella (3)**. The knee joint is a pivotal hinge joint, in which flexion and extension is possible, as well as rotating movements.

Structure   The patella is enclosed as a sesamoid bone in the **patellar tendon (Lig. patellae, 4)**, the terminal ligament of the M. quadriceps femoris. The femoral condyles wind onto the tibial condyles with increasing flexion, so that when extending, their flatter, anterior portions lie on the tibia. When flexing, their more kyphotic posterior portions lie on the tibia.

Femoral and tibial condyles are not congruent. To offset this incongruity, two fibrocartilaginous wedges, the menisci, form part of the knee joint. Both menisci are attached to the knee joint capsule. The **lateral meniscus (Meniscus lateralis, 5)** is more circular, while the **medial meniscus (Meniscus medialis, 6)** forms a C-opening inwards. When seen ventrally, one can see the **medial (1a)** and **lateral (1b) femoral condyle** as well as the **medial (2a)** and **lateral (2b) tibial condyle**.

Ligaments   The knee joint capsule is strengthened with ligaments:
- outer ligaments, incl.
  - **Lig. patellae (4)**
  - **Ligg. collateralia fibulare and tibiale (7)**
- inner ligaments
  - **Lig. cruciatum anterius (anterior cruciate ligament, 9)**
  - **Lig. cruciatum posterius (posterior cruciate ligament, 10)**

Laterally and medially, the Ligg. collateralia straddle the knee joint.

The **Lig. collaterale tibiale (7)** runs from the Epicondylus medialis to the **femur (1a),** to the medial edge of the tibia. The Lig. collaterale tibiale is attached to the medial meniscus and thus lessens its movement.

The **Lig. collaterale fibulare** (not shown) runs from the Epicondylus lateralis of the femur to the **Caput fibulae (8)** and has no contact to the knee joint capsule.

Both the collateral ligaments are tight when stretched and slack when flexing. Thereby rotation movements are only possible when the knee is flexed. The collateral ligaments largely inhibit passive abduction and adduction movements in the knee joint. Both the **Ligg. cruciata genus (cruciate ligaments)** can be seen in the Fossa intercondylaris.

The **Lig. cruciatum anterius (9)** runs from the posterior, inner surface of the lateral femoral condyle to the Area intercondylaris anterior of the tibia. It runs from above, the outside and the posterior to below, the inside and the anterior.

The **Lig. cruciatum posterius (10)** comes from the anterior, inner surface of the medial femoral condyle and runs to the Area intercondylaris posterior of the tibia. It runs from the anterior, above and inside to the posterior, below and outside. In this way, both cruciate ligaments are wound around each other. The cruciate ligaments are partially tight in all positions of the knee joint and thereby provide important protection for the joint. Parts of the cruciate ligaments thereby inhibit almost every movement in the knee joint. With the inner rotation, the cruciate ligaments wind around each other more tightly.

Clinical remarks

Injuries to the meniscus mostly relate to the medial meniscus. It is less flexible because it is attached to the Lig. collaterale tibiale and it can tear with outwards rotation trauma in a flexed position. The poor regenerative capacity of the cartilaginous tissue then often needs the meniscus to be partially or fully removed. In turn, this can lead to a further attrition of the joint cartilage.

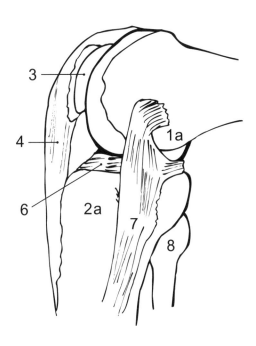

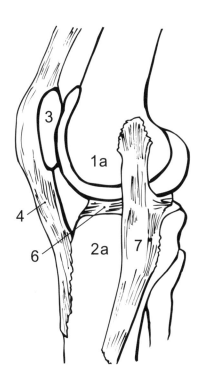

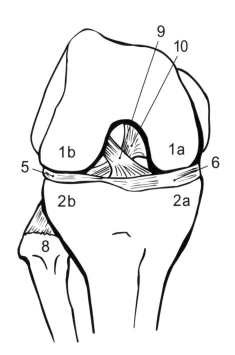

Abb. 3.5

3.6 Calf muscles

The calf muscles are flexors for the ankle joints. They are divided into:
- a superficial layer
- a deep layer

Superficial layer   The superficial layer of the calf muscles constitute the **M. triceps surae**. It consists of:
- the **M. gastrocnemius (1)**
- the **M. soleus (2)**

The **M. gastrocnemius (1)** originates with its Caput mediale proximally of the medial femoral condyle, with its Caput laterale proximal of the lateral femoral condyle.

The **M. soleus (2)** originates from the head of the fibula and from the tibia. The gap between both the points of origin is straddled by a tendinous arch, the **Arcus tendineus musculi solei (2a)**.

Both muscles unite into a common terminal tendon, the **Achilles tendon (Tendo calcaneus, 3)**. This attaches at the Tuber calcanei.

The M. triceps surae functions as a plantar flexor and supinator of the foot. The **M. gastrocnemius** also flexes in the knee joint.

Deep layer   The deep layer of the calf muscles can be seen after removal of the M. triceps surae:
- **M. flexor digitorum longus (4)**
- **M. tibialis posterior (5)**
- **M. flexor hallucis longus (6)**
- **M. popliteus (7)**

The **M. flexor digitorum longus (4)** originates furthest medially from the dorsal tibia distal of the M. soleus. It runs behind the **Malleolus medialis (8)** to the sole of the foot and ends there at the base of the distal phalanges II–V. The M. flexor digitorum longus induces a plantar flexion and supination of the foot and flexes the toes II–V.

The **M. tibialis posterior (5)** originates from the Membrana interossea cruris and the adjoining parts of the tibia and fibula. It crosses the tendons of the M. flexor digitorum longus below the distal lower leg and thereby forms the **Chiasma cruris (9)**. It attaches at the Tuberositas ossis navicularis and at the Os cuneiforme mediale. The M. tibialis posterior supinates the foot and induces a light plantar flexion.

The **M. flexor hallucis longus (6)** originates from the Membrana interossea cruris and the fibula. It runs to the sole of the foot and attaches there to the distal phalanx of the big toe. The M.

flexor hallucis longus flexes the big toe and induces plantar flexion and supination of the foot.

The **M. popliteus (7)** can be seen above the **Arcus tendineus musculi solei (2a)**. It originates from the Condylus lateralis of the femur and attaches above the Linea poplitea of the tibia. The M. popliteus spans the dorsal knee joint capsule and thereby prevents it from locking.

Note

Innervation
Calf muscles → N. tibialis

Clinical remarks

Because of degenerative changes, the Achilles tendon can tear with excessive strain of the M. triceps surae (e.g. in sport). The patient is then no longer able to stand on their toes.

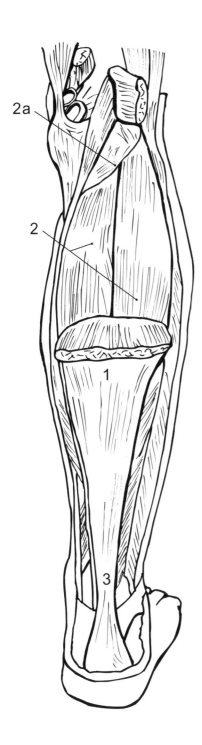

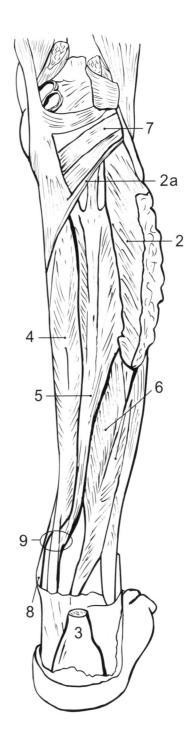

Abb. 3.6

3.7 Extensors and the peroneal muscle group of the lower leg

The muscles of the lower leg are divided into the:
- extensors,
- peroneal group
- flexors (➤ Chap. 3.6)

Extensors   The following belong to the extensors of the lower leg:
- **M. tibialis anterior (1)**
- **M. extensor digitorum longus (2)**
- **M. peroneus [fibularis] tertius (3)**
- **M. extensor hallucis longus (4)**

The **M. tibialis anterior (1)** originates from the lateral surface of the tibia and the Membrana interossea cruris. Its tendon passes under the **Retinacula musculorum extensorum (5)** to the Os cuneiforme mediale and to the Os metatarsale I. The M. tibialis anterior induces a dorsal flexion and a weak supination of the foot.

The **M. extensor digitorum longus (2)** originates from the Condylus lateralis tibiae, from the front of the fibula and the Membrana interossea cruris. Its tendon runs below the Retinacula musculorum extensorum and then divides into four terminal tendons, which radiate into the dorsal aponeuroses of the toes II–V. The M. extensor digitorum longus enables dorsal extension and pronation of the foot. As the 5th tendon, it splits away from the **M. peroneus [fibularis] tertius (3)**, which inserts at the Os metatarsale V.

At its point of origin on the middle fibula and the Membrana interossea cruris, the **M. extensor hallucis longus (4)** is hidden by the M. tibialis posterior and M. extensor digitorum longus. Its tendon becomes visible at the distal lower leg and runs to the basis of the end phalanx of the big toe. Its function is to dorsally flex the foot and to extend the base of the big toe and distal joint.

Peroneal group   The **M. peroneus [fibularis] longus (6)** originates from the head and upper shaft of the fibula and from the Septa intermuscularia anterius and posterius, which confine the peroneal compartment. Its tendon runs behind the **Malleolus lateralis (7)** below the **Retinacula musculorum peroneorum [fibularium] (8)**, bends at the lateral margin of the sole of the foot and runs obliquely below the sole of the foot to the Os metatarsale I and Os cuneiforme mediale. The M. peroneus [fibularis] longus induces pronation and plantar flexion

of the foot. Running across the bottom of the sole of the foot, it spans the transverse arch of the foot.

The **M. peroneus [fibularis] brevis (9)** originates from the distal part of the fibula and inserts at the Tuberositas ossis metatarsalis V. Its function is the pronation and plantar flexion of the foot.

Note

Innervation

Extensors → N. peroneus [fibularis] profundus
Peroneal group → N. peroneus [fibularis] superficialis

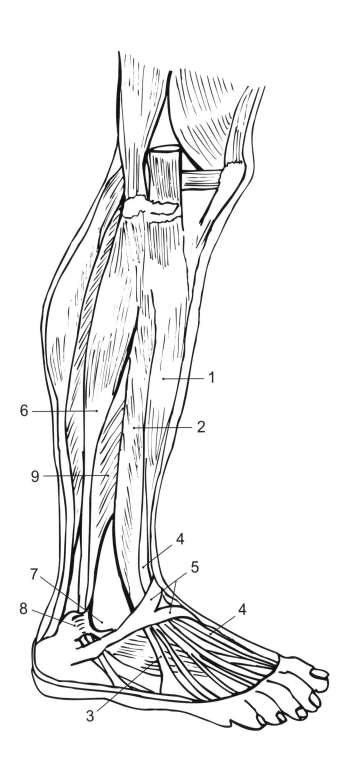

Abb. 3.7

3.8 Upper ankle joint (Articulatio talocruralis)

Structure   The upper ankle joint is a **hinge joint,** in which the foot can be flexed plantar (i.e. with the toes flexing down towards the sole of the foot) or dorsally, with the toes extending backwards. The upper ankle joint consists of the distal end of the tibia (shin, 1) and the fibula (calfbone, 2) as well as the talus (ankle bone, 3).

- The **Malleolus medialis** of the **tibia (1a)** and the **Malleolus lateralis of the Fibula (2a)** form the **malleolus,** which forms the joint socket of the upper ankle joint. Thereby the Malleolus lateralis (external malleolus) extends further distally. At its distal end, the tibia and fibula are tightly connected to each other via the **Ligamenta tibiofibulare anterius (4)** and **posterius (5)**. They are also described as anterior and posterior syndesmosis.
- The joint head of the upper ankle joint forms the **Trochlea tali (3a)** .

Ligaments   The upper ankle joint is medially as well as laterally secured by numerous ligaments:

- Medially, four partial ligaments can be seen, running from the Malleolus medialis to the metatarsal bone, and which can also be described in its entirety as the **deltoid ligament (Lig. deltoideum)**: the **Pars tibiotalaris anterior (6)** and **posterior (7)** run to the medial neck of the talus. The **Pars tibionavicularis (8)** runs to the Os naviculare (scaphoid bone) and the **Pars tibiocalcanea (9)** to the **calcaneus (10)**.
- The three lateral ligaments run from the Malleolus lateralis to the talus and the calcaneus. The **Ligamenta talofibulare anterius (11)** and **posterius** (not shown) are shown, as well as the **Ligamentum calcaneofibulare (12)**.

Clinical remarks

Despite being secured with these ligaments, turning the ankle with the lateral **(supination injury)** or medial margin of the foot **(pronation injury)** leads to distortion (spraining) of the upper ankle joint. With supination trauma, the lateral ligaments are affected in the injury, and with pronation trauma, the medial. Depending on the extent and the type of trauma, injury to the ligament connections between the distal tibia and fibula (tear of the syndesmosis) or bony structures (e.g. fracture of the Malleolus medialis) or a fracture of the fibula at various levels can result.

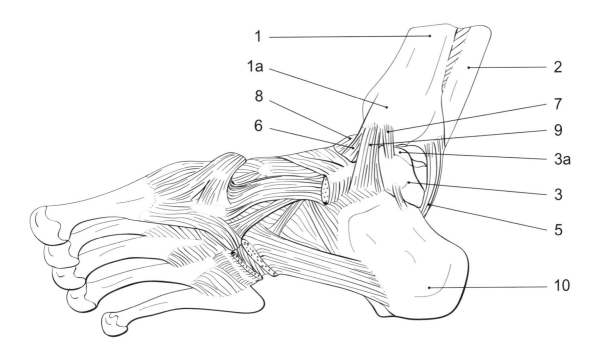

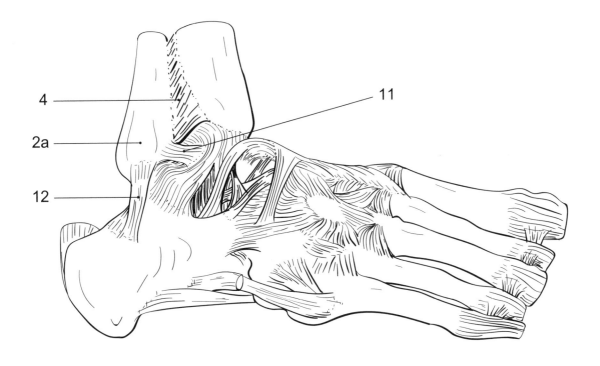

Abb. 3.8

3.9 The instep

On the instep, the extensor tendons on the lower leg and the muscles of the instep are visible.

Extensors of the lower leg   The tendons of the **M. tibialis anterior** (1) run below the Retinaculum musculorum extensorum superius, then through the medial compartment below the **Retinaculum musculorum extensorum inferius** (2) to the Os cuneiforme mediale and the Os metatarsale I.

The tendon of the **M. extensor hallucis longus** (3) runs through the middle compartment below the **Retinaculum musculorum extensorum inferius** (2) and inserts at the base of the distal phalanx of the big toe.

The tendon of the **M. extensor digitorum longus** (4) runs through the lateral compartment below the Retinaculum musculorum extensorum inferius (2), divides into four terminal tendons and radiates into the **dorsal aponeurosis** (5) of the toes II–V. Splitting away, the tendon of the **M. peroneus [fibularis] tertius** (6) runs to the base of the Os metatarsale V.

Muscles of the instep   On the instep, the **M. extensor digitorum brevis** (7) and the **M. extensor hallucis brevis** (8) are visible. Both muscles originate from the calcaneus and radiate together with the long extensors into the dorsal aponeurosis of the toes. Thereby the 5th toe often does not retain a tendon. The M. extensor digitorum brevis and the M. extensor hallucis brevis are innervated by the N. fibularis profundus. They extend the toes.

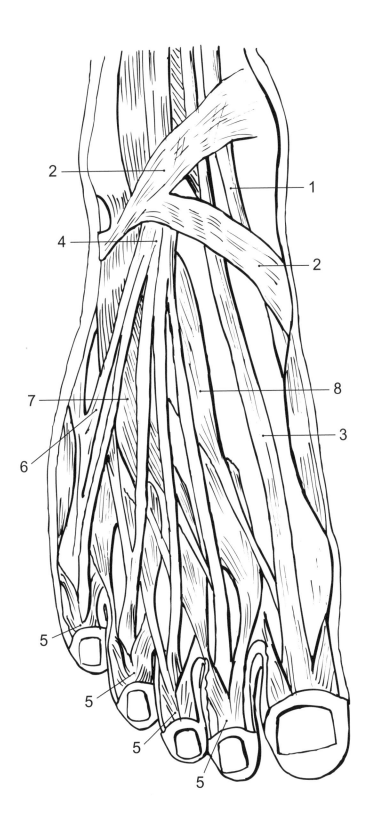

Abb. 3.9

3.10 Sole of the foot

The muscles of the sole of the foot can be divided into:
- a superficial layer of muscles
- muscles of the ball of the big toe
- muscles of the ball of the little toe

Superficial layer of muscles When dissecting the **plantar aponeurosis (1)**, the muscles and tendons of the sole of the foot become visible.

The most superficial layer is formed by the **M. flexor digitorum brevis (2)**. In the illustration on the right, it has been partially removed and folded back dorsally. It originates from the Tuber calcanei, attaches to the middle phalanges of the toes II-V with four furcate tendons and flexes the middle phalanges of these toes. Below the M. flexor digitorum brevis one can see the tendons of the long flexors of the lower leg. They reach the sole of the foot behind the Malleolus medialis and below the muscles of the ball of the big toe.

Because the **M. flexor hallucis longus (3)** originates further laterally on the lower leg, (➤ Chap. 3.6), but inserts further medially on the foot than the **M. flexor digitorum longus (4)**, its tendon crosses that of the M. flexor digitorum longus and thereby forms the **Chiasma plantare (5)**.

The **M. flexor hallucis longus (3)** attaches to the distal phalanx of the big toe.

The four tendons of the **M. flexor digitorum longus (4)** insert on the distal phalanges of the toes II–V. Thereby they penetrate the tendons of the **M. flexor digitorum brevis (2a)**.

The **M. quadratus plantae (6)** originates from the Tuber calcanei. It radiates into the distal tendons of the M. flexor digitorum longus and thereby changes it transversely to run in a sagittal direction.

Muscles of the ball of the big toe The **M. abductor hallucis (7)** originates from the Proc. medialis of the Tuber calcanei and attaches to the medial sesamoid bone and to the proximal phalanx on the big toe. It abducts the big toe.

The **M. flexor hallucis brevis (8)** originates from the Os cuneiforme I and attaches to the proximal phalanx and to the lateral sesamoid bone of the big toe. It flexes the big toe.

Muscles of the ball of the little toe The **M. flexor digiti minimi brevis (9)** originates from the base of the Os metatarsale V and inserts at the proximal phalanx of the little toe. It flexes the little toe.

The **M. abductor digiti minimi (10)** originates from the Proc. lateralis of the Tuber calcanei and attaches to the proximal phalanx of the little toe. It flexes the little toe.

Deep down, laterally of the M. flexor digitorum brevis, the tendon of the **M. peroneus [fibularis] longus (11)** can be seen where it emerges from the lateral margin of the foot, spans the sole of the foot and inserts at the Os cuneiforme mediale. In this way this tendon serves to dynamically stabilize the transverse arch of the foot.

Note

Innervation

Muscles of the sole of the foot → Nn. plantares mediales and laterales from the N. tibialis

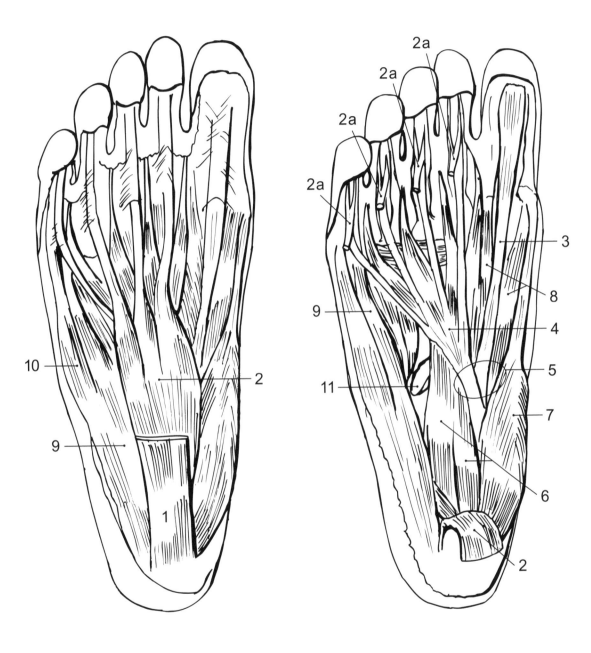

Abb. 3.10

53

3.11 Pathways in the Trigonum femorale

The Trigonum femorale is located on the proximal, ventral upper leg. It is bounded by:
- the **Lig. inguinale (1)**
- the **M. sartorius (2)**
- the **M. adductor longus (3)**

The **M. pectineus (4)** and the **M. iliopsoas (5)** form its base.
The **M. iliopsoas (5)** originates through the merging of the M. psoas, which arises from the lower thoracic and lumbar vertebrae, with the **M. iliacus (6)**, which arises from the Ala ossis ilii. Together they run below the Lig. inguinale through the Lacuna musculorum to the upper leg and attach to the Trochanter minor. The M. iliopsoas is the most important flexor in the hip joint. It is innervated directly by the Plexus lumbalis and by the **N. femoralis (7)**. The N. femoralis runs together with the M. iliopsoas through the Lacuna musculorum into the Trigonum femorale and there divides into its muscular branches (Rr. musculares) for the Mm. sartorius and quadriceps femoris, and into the cutaneous branches (Rr. cutanei) for the ventral upper leg.
Further medially in the Trigonum femorale are the **A. femoralis (8)** and the **V. femoralis (9)**. Together with the **R. femoralis of the N. genitofemoralis** (not shown), they arrive at the Trigonum femorale through the Lacuna vasorum.
The **A. femoralis (8)** here provides the **A. profunda femoris (10)**, of which the branches supply the adductors and the dorsal side of the upper leg. The A. femoralis itself runs distally below the M. sartorius and then moves into the Canalis adductorius, which is bounded by the **M. vastus medialis (11)** as well as the **Mm. adductores longus (3)** and **magnus** (not shown). Following this pathway, it ends up in the Fossa poplitea (➤ Chap. 3.13).
The **V. femoralis (9)** is located furthest medially in the Trigonum femorale. Here it incorporates numerous epifascial veins, incl. the **V. saphena magna (12)**.

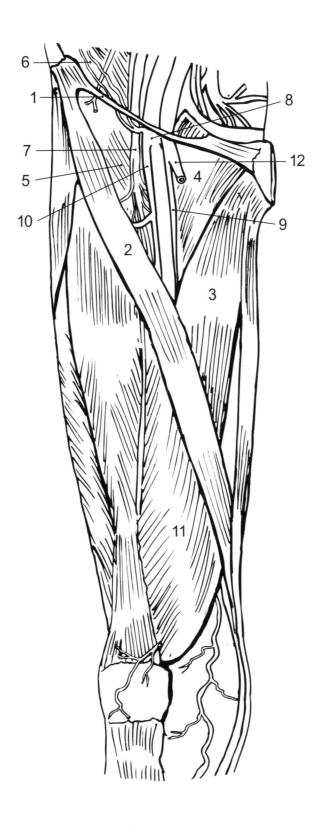

Abb. 3.11

55

3.12 The gluteal area

The key gluteal areas (Regio glutealis) are:
- the Crista iliaca
- the anal cleft
- the M. tensor fasciae latae
- the gluteal fold

The pathways of the gluteal area come from the inner pelvis and leave it via the Foramina supra- and infrapiriforme.

Foramen suprapiriforme Cranial of the **M. piriformis (1)**, the **A. glutea superior (2)** moves out of the pelvis into the gluteal area. It is a parietal branch of the A. iliaca interna and supplies the **Mm. glutei medius (3)** and **minimus** (not shown). Together with the artery, the **N. gluteus superior** (not shown) runs out of the Plexus sacralis. It branches out into the Mm. glutei medius and minimus and innervates them.

Foramen infrapiriforme Caudally of the **M. piriformis (1),** the **N. gluteus inferior (4)** leaves the pelvis, together with its eponymous artery. The nerve innervates the M. gluteus maximus.

The **A. glutea inferior (5)** is a parietal branch of the A. iliaca interna and supplies extensive portions of the gluteal area.

The **N. ischiadicus (6)** also reaches the gluteal area via the Foramen infrapiriforme. It originates from the Plexus sacralis and either leaves via the Foramen infrapiriforme, already split into two branches, or splits further along its route in the dorsal upper leg into the **N. tibialis (7)** and the **N. peroneus [fibularis] communis (8)**. Both branches innervate the ischiocrural mucles on the upper leg:
- **M. semimembranosus (9)**
- **M. semitendinosus (10)**
- **M. biceps femoris (11)**

The **N. cutaneus femoris posterior (12)** is a sensory cutaneous nerve which innervates the dorsal side of the upper leg.

The **A. pudenda interna (13)** is a visceral branch of the A. iliaca interna. The A. pudenda interna and the **N. pudendus (14)** from the Plexus sacralis bend around the Spina ischiadica immediately after leaving the Foramen infrapiriforme and re-enter the pelvis via the Foramen ischiadicum minus. There they reach the Fossa ischioanalis and supply the pelvic floor and the outer genitalia.

Clinical remarks

Intramuscular (IM) injections are often administered, in the gluteal area e.g., vaccinations. It is important to administer the injection in the outer, upper quarter of the gluteal area, i.e. in the area of the M. gluteus medius. The correct injection site can be ascertained with the help of the **Hochstetter pinch method**. An incorrectly placed injection in the middle of the gluteal area can hit the N. ischiadicus. Oily vaccines can, in particular, cause permanent damage to the N. peroneus [fibularis] communis, causing a peroneal paralysis with malfunction of the extensors on the lower leg and clinical presentation of a drop-foot gait.

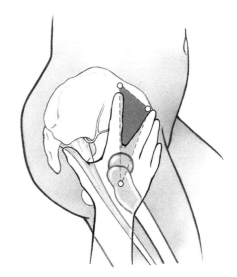

Abb. 3.12 **Hochstetter pinch method.** Injecting between the index and middle fingers.

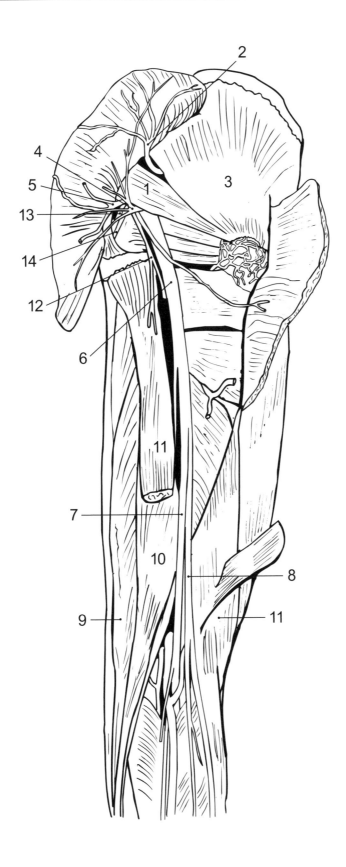

Abb. 3.13

3.13 Pathways of the Fossa poplitea

The Fossa poplitea (back of the knee) is a rhomboid space, confined cranially and caudally by muscles.

- Two muscles of the Pes anserinus superficialis, the **Mm. gracilis (1)** and the **semitendinosus (2),** as well as the **M. semimembranosus (3)**, constitute the cranial medial borders of the Fossa poplitea.
- The **M. biceps femoris (4)** is located cranially laterally.
- Both the heads of the **M. gastrocnemius (5)** can be seen caudally.

Blood Vessel supply The **A. poplitea (6)** is located furthest medially in the Fossa poplitea. It arises from the A. femoralis, which reaches the back of the knee via the Canalis adductorius. The A. poplitea provides branches here for the knee joint and for the flexors on the proximal lower leg.

The **V. poplitea (7)** is located laterally of the A. poplitea. It originates from the confluence of the deep lower leg veins and continues in the Canalis adductorius in the V. femoralis. In the Fossa poplitea it incorporates the epifascial **V. saphena parva (8)**.

Nerves The **N. tibialis (9)** and the **N. peroneus [fibularis] communis (10)** are located furthest laterally. The N. tibialis descends further into the flexor compartment of the lower leg. At the back of the knee, it provides the **N. cutaneus surae medialis (11)** as a cutaneous branch for the calf. The N. peroneus [fibularis] communis then turns to the fibula. It winds itself around the head of the fibula and splits into two branches, the **Nn. peronei superficialis** and **profundus**. At the back of the knee, it provides a cutaneous branch for the calf, the **N. cutaneus surae lateralis (12)**.

Clinical remarks

The N. peroneus [fibularis] communis is vulnerable to **fractures of the head of the fibula** as it runs very superficially in this area. Besides loss of sensitivity in the lower leg and the instep, lesions of the nerve cause malfunction of the extensors and the peroneal group in the lower leg.

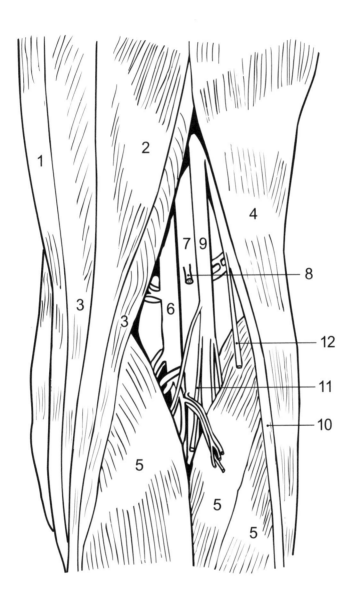

Abb. 3.14

3.14 Pathways of the extensors and peroneal compartments of the lower leg

There are three muscle compartments on the lower leg:
- the extensor compartment
- the flexor compartment (➤ Chap. 3.15)
- the peroneal compartment

Nerves of the extensors and peroneal compartments   The **N. peroneus [fibularis] communis (1)** runs around the Caput fibulae and, in the peroneal compartment, divides into its terminal branches, the **N. peroneus [fibularis] superficialis (2)** and the **N. peroneus [fibularis] profundus (3)**.

The **N. peroneus [fibularis] superficialis (2)** continues in the peroneal compartment and here innervates the **Mm. peronei longus (4)** and **brevis (5)**.

The **N. peroneus [fibularis] profundus (3)** penetrates the Septum intermusculare cruris anterius and thereby ends up in the extensor compartment of the lower leg. There it innervates the **Mm. tibialis anterior (6), extensor hallucis longus (7)** and **extensor digitorum longus (8)**.

Arterial supply   The **A. tibialis anterior (9)** moves through the Membrana interossea cruris of the Fossa poplitea in the extensor compartment. There it runs laterally from the **M. tibialis anterior (6)** and supplies the muscles of the extensor compartment. Its terminal branch, the **A. dorsalis pedis (10)**, runs along the instep laterally of the **tendon of the M. extensor hallucis longus (7a)**, supplies the toes and communicates with the Arcus plantaris (➤ Chap. 3.17) via an R. profundus (not shown).

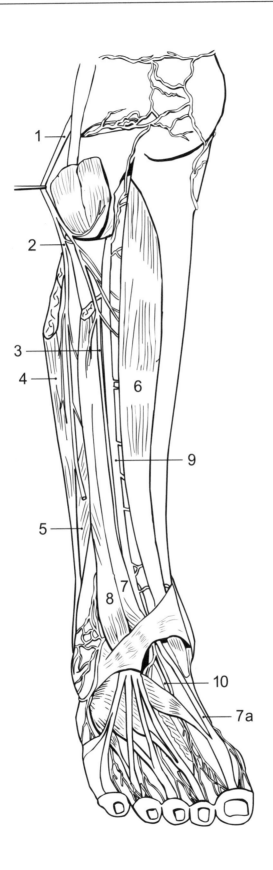

Abb. 3.15

61

3.15 Pathways of the flexor compartment of the lower leg

On the lower leg there are three muscle compartments:
- the extensor compartment, (➤ Chap. 3.14)
- the flexor compartment
- the peroneal compartment (➤ Chap. 3.14)

With removal of the superficial layer of the flexors (**Mm. gastrocnemius, 1** and **soleus, 2**), the pathways of the flexor compartment become visible.

Arterial supply   Along its course, the **A. poplitea (3)** splits away from the Fossa poplitea, below the **Arcus tendineus musculi solei (4)** and into the flexor compartment, forming its terminal branches:
- The **A. tibialis anterior** (not shown) runs ventrally into the extensor compartment.
- The **A. tibialis posterior (5)** runs distally between the superficial and the deep flexors and behind the Malleolus medialis to the sole of the foot.

The **A. fibularis** (not shown) exits from the proximal lower leg, also running distally in the flexor compartment, hidden by the **M. flexor hallucis longus (6),** to the **Malleolus lateralis (7).**

Nerves   The **N. tibialis (8)** which originates from the Fossa poplitea, runs below the Arcus musculi solei in the flexor compartment and continues alongside the A. tibialis posterior to the **Malleolus medialis (9).**

Clinical remarks

During a physical examination, the condition of the arteries can be checked by palpating the **pulse of the foot**. This can be done in areas such as behind the **Malleolus medialis (9),** where the pulse of the A. tibialis posterior is palpable.

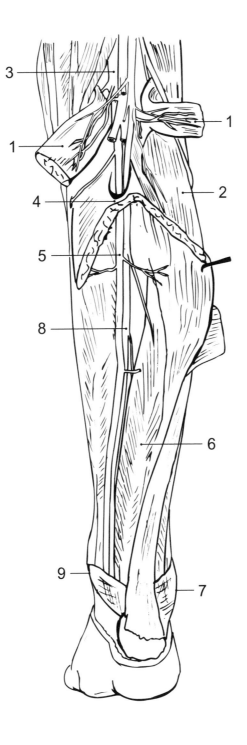

Abb. 3.16

63

3.16 Pathways of the instep

The epifascial pathways of the distal lower leg and the instep can be seen on the illustration.

Venous supply   On the medial instep, the **V. marginalis medialis (1)** is visible and continues at the **Malleolus medialis (2)** in the **V. saphena magna (3)** . This large vein then runs epifascially along the medial side of the lower and upper leg and flows into the subfascial **V. femoralis** only once it is in the area of the Trigonum femorale.

The **V. marginalis lateralis (4)** runs along the lateral margin of the foot. It continues at the **Malleolus lateralis (5)** in the V. saphena parva. This epifascial vein then runs on the dorsal side of the lower leg and flows into the **V. poplitea** in the area of the Fossa poplitea.

Nerves   In the area of the distal lower leg, on the fibular side, the **N. peroneus [fibularis] superficialis (6)** leaves the peroneal compartment via the Fascia cruris and moves to the surface. It splits into the **Nn. cutanei dorsales intermedius (7)** and **medialis (8),** which innervate the skin of the instep and the dorsal side of the toes.

The **N. peroneus [fibularis] profundus (9)** penetrates the fascia between the 1st and 2nd metatarsal bones in the area of the midfoot. It splits into the **Nn. digitales dorsales I and II (10),** which innervates the skin between the 1st and 2nd toes.

The terminal branches of the **N. saphenus (11)** can be seen at the **Malleolus medialis (2),** adjacent to the **V. saphena magna (3)**. This terminal branch of the N. femoralis innervates the skin at the medial lower leg up to the Malleolus medialis.

On the distal lower leg, the **N. cutaneus surae medialis (12)** emerging from the N. tibialis can be seen on the tibial side.

The lateral margin of the foot innervates the **N. cutaneus dorsalis lateralis (13)** from the N. suralis.

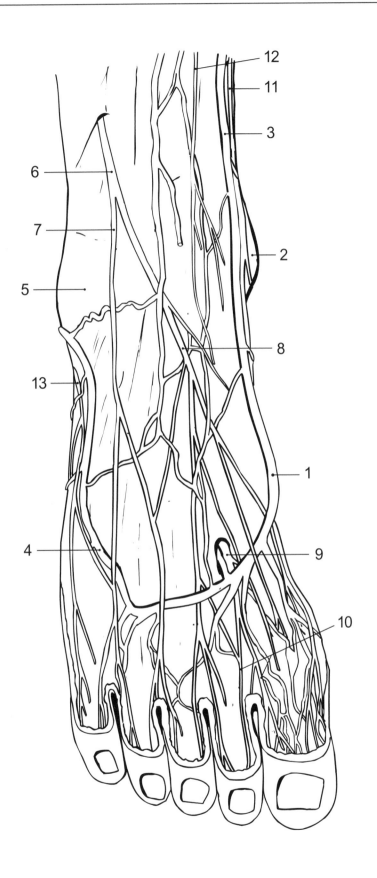

Abb. 3.17

3.17 Pathways of the sole of the foot

The pathways of the sole of the foot are visible after removing parts of the plantar aponeurosis (1) and of the M. flexor digitorum brevis (2).

Arterial supply Below the origin of the **M. abductor hallucis (3),** the **A. tibialis posterior,** which arises from the flexor compartment of the lower leg, splits into its terminal branches:

- The **A. plantaris lateralis (4)** runs between the **M. flexor digitorum brevis (2)** and the **M. quadratus plantae (5)** to the lateral sole of the foot. At the level of the base of the Os metatarsale V, **Arcus plantaris profundus (6)** turns to medial. From the Arcus plantaris profundus, the **Aa. metatarsales plantares (7)** run to the toes. The Arcus plantaris profundus anastomoses with the R. plantaris profundus of the A. dorsalis pedis ($\succ$ Chap. 3.14).
- The **A. plantaris medialis (8)** is at first hidden on its course between the Mm. abductor and the Flexor hallucis brevis. It provides a **R. profundus (8a)** to the **Arcus plantaris profundus (6)** and a **R. superficialis (8b)** to the medial margin of the big toe.

Nerves Below the origin of the **M. abductor hallucis (3),** the **N. tibialis,** arising from the flexor compartment of the lower leg, splits into its terminal branches:

- The **N. plantaris medialis (9)** is located between the M. abductor hallucis and the M. flexor digitorum brevis. It provides a medial branch to the medial margin of the big toe and a lateral branch. The lateral branch splits into the Nn. digitales plantares communes, which provide the **Nn. digitales plantares proprii (10)** to the 1st to 4th toes.
- The **N. plantaris lateralis (11)** runs in the Sulcus plantaris lateralis alongside the ball of the little toe. It provides the branches to the muscles of the ball of the little toe and splits into an **R. profundus (11a)** and an **R. superficialis (11b).** The **R. profundus** innervates the Mm. interossei, the fibular Mm. lumbricales, the **M. adductor hallucis (12)** and the **Caput laterale of the M. flexor hallucis brevis (13).** The **R. superficialis** constitutes the **N. digitalis plantaris communis IV (14),** which provides the **Nn. digitales plantares proprii (10)** to the 4th and 5th toes.

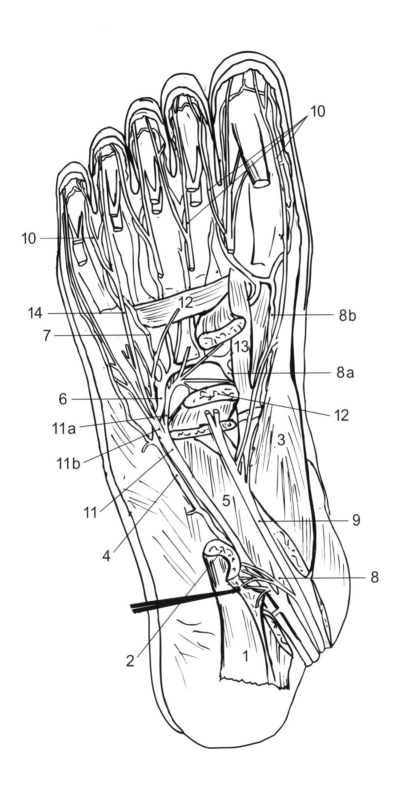

Abb. 3.18

67

3.18 Plexus sacralis

The Plexus sacralis is formed by the **Rami anteriores (1)** of the spinal nerves L4–S3. It is hidden by the M. piriformis on the back and lateral walls of the lesser pelvis on the Facies pelvica of the Os sacrum. To help with orientation, the vertebral body has been marked with LIV–SV. The Plexus sacralis provides the following branches:

- The **N. gluteus superior (2)** originates from the spinal cord segments L4–S1. It leaves the pelvis via the Foramen suprapiriforme and ends up between the Mm. glutei medius and minimus, which it also innervates.
- The **N. gluteus inferior (3)** from the spinal cord segments L5–S2 passes through the Foramen infrapiriforme and innervates the M. gluteus maximus.
- The **N. cutaneus femoris posterior (4)** from the spinal cord segments S1–S3 also passes through the Foramen infrapiriforme and comes to the surface at the lower margin of the M. gluteus maximus. Here it provides the Nn. clunium inferiores, which also sensorily innervate the skin of the gluteal area. The N. cutaneus femoris posterior itself innervates the skin on the dorsal side of the upper leg.
- The **N. ischiadicus (5)** from the spinal cord segments L4–S3 penetrates the Foramen infrapiriforme. It runs to distal and splits into the **N. tibialis (6)** and the **N. peroneus [fibularis] communis (7)** at a variable level. Both innervate the ischiocrural muscles on the upper leg. The **N. tibialis** runs through the Fossa poplitea in the flexor compartment of the lower leg. Here it innervates the flexors, and its terminal branches, the **Nn. plantares medialis and lateralis,** run to the sole of the foot. The **N. peroneus [fibularis] communis** winds itself around the head of the fibula and then splits into its terminal branches, the **N. peroneus [fibularis] superficialis** to the Mm. peronei longus and brevis and the **N. peroneus [fibularis] profundus** to the extensors of the lower leg and the instep.

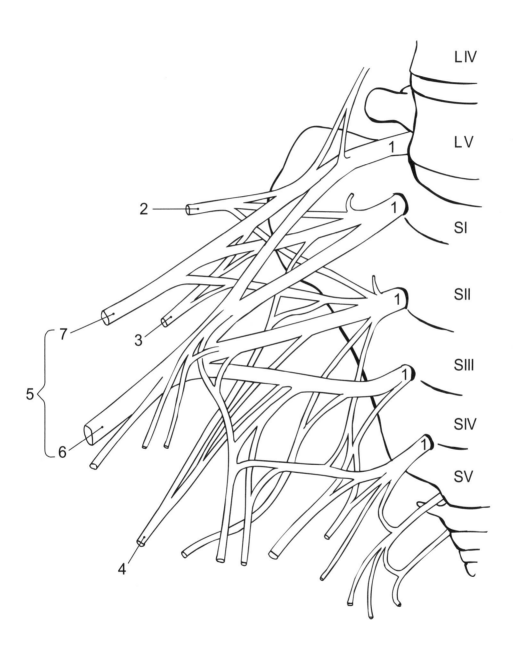

LIV

LV

SI

SII

SIII

SIV

SV

Abb. 3.19

4.1 Thoracic organs in situ

Serous cavities in the thorax   The serous cavities of the thorax are visible after removing the sternum and the ventral sections of the ribs.
The following can be differentiated:
- the right and left **pleural cavity**, which contains the lungs, as well as
- the **pericardial cavity**, which contains the heart

The serosa, which coats these serous cavities, consists of two membranes: the **visceral membrane (Pleura visceralis and/or epicardium)** is located directly on the organs, and the **parietal membrane (Pleura parietalis and/or pericardium)** covers the inner surface of the body cavities. The Pleura parietalis is divided into the following parts:
- the **Pars mediastinalis**, which covers the mediastinum and the **pericardium (1)**
- the **Pars costalis (costal pleura, 2a)**, which covers the sternum, ribs and the vertebral body
- the **Pars diaphragmatica (2b)**, which covers the surface of the diaphragm

Between the two membranes of the serosa is a capillary cavity, which is filled with serous fluid and which allows the membranes to slide against each other. This cavity facilitates movement of the heart in the pericardium and/or the movement of the lungs during inspiration and expiration (pleural space).

Expansion of the pleural cavities   In the illustration, both the pleural cavities have been exposed by removing the the ventral sections of the **parietal pleura,** and the **lungs (3a and b)** are visible.
The pleural cavities with the **pleura dome (4a and b)** reach into the Fossa supraclavicularis major in the area of the neck. From the pleural dome, the medial borders of both the pleural cavities converge, until they almost touch each other at the point where the 2nd–4th ribs attach. This area is known as the **Septum pleurae (5)**. Cranial of the Septum pleurae there is a triangular area known as the Trigonum thymicum. This is filled by the **thymus (6)** which is adjacent to the ventral thoracic wall. Caudal to the Septum pleurae, the borders of the two pleural cavities again diverge. On the right side, the pleural border deviates from the median at the point where the 6th rib attaches and then descends obliquely. With every anatomical line (midclavicular line, anterior axillary line, etc.) the pleural border moves deeper by approx. one intercostal space, so that it reaches the level of the 12th rib in the area of the paravertebral line on the back.

As the apex of the heart points to the left and correspondingly occupies more space than on the right, the pleural border on the left already deviates from the median at the point where the 4th ribs attach. From the anterior axillary line on the left, it then still takes the same course as described above for the right side. As both the pleural cavities diverge caudally from the Septum pleurae, a triangular area between them is left hollow, in which a part of the **pericardium (1)** lies directly next to the ventral thoracic wall. This area is therefore known as the Trigonum pericardiacum. The biggest part of the pericardium is however covered with both the pleural cavities, and is therefore not visible here.

Lungs   By opening the costal Pleura parietalis, the lungs become visible. They both respectively extend with an **apex (Apex pulmonis, 7a and b)** into the **pleural dome (4a and b)**, but without filling the pleural cavities completely. The borders of the lungs have a similar pathway to the pleural borders described above, but approx. two intercostal spaces further cranially. Thereby the **Recessus costomediastinalis (8)** develops between the mediastinal and the costal Pleura parietalis, as well as the **Recessus costodiaphragmaticus (9)** between the costal and diaphragmatic Pleura parietalis. The lungs can expand with inspiration in this recess of the pleural cavity.The **upper lobe (Lobus superior, 10a)** and the **middle lobe (Lobus medius, 11)**, are visible, pointing to the ventral thoracic wall in the area of the right lung. Ventrally on the left, the **upper lobe (Lobus superior, 10b)** can be seen. On both sides, the **lower lobe (Lobus inferior, 12a und b)** is broadly facing dorsolaterally and is therefore hardly visible from this side.
The lobes of the lungs are separated from each other with deep fissures: with the right and left lung, the **Fissura obliqua (13a and b)** sections off a lower lobe, and additionally with the right lung, the **Fissura horizontalis (14)** separates the upper lobe from the middle lobe.

Clinical remarks

The pleural cavities extend with the pleural dome into the Fossa supraclavicularis major and are there positioned directly adjacent to the veins near the heart (Vv. subclaviae, Vv. brachiocephalicae). By placing a central catheter in these veins, the pleural dome can accidentally be punctured, letting air into the pleural space. This can lead to a **pneumothorax,** i.e. the visceral and parietal pleura no longer work together and the lungs collapse.

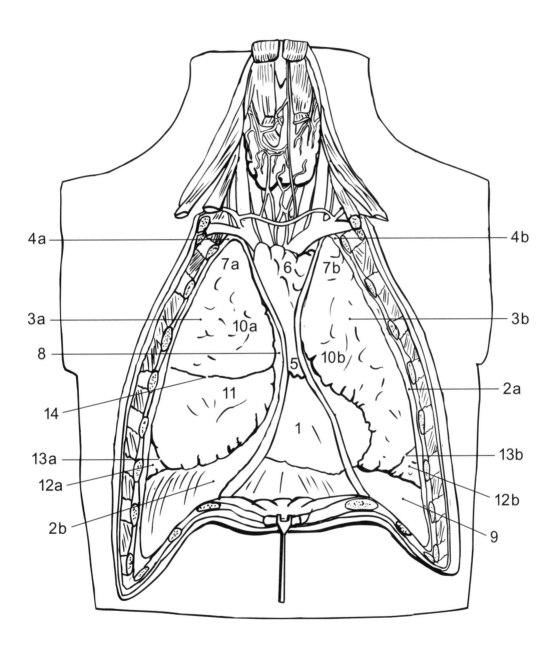

4a — — 4b

7a 6 7b

3a — 3b

8 —

10a

10b

5

14 — 11 — 2a

13a — — 13b

12a —

2b — 12b

1

9

Abb. 4.1

71

4.2 Heart

The heart has the shape of an upside-down cone. It faces upwards to the right, while its **apex cordis (1)** faces downwards and to the left. The surface of the heart is covered by a visceral serous membrane, the epicardium. The epicardium extends up to the large vessels near the heart. There this membrane turns back over itself and becomes the parietal membrane, the **pericardium (2)**, forming the pericardial sac.

Ventral view   In the ventral view, one can see the **Facies sternocostalis (3)** of the heart. It is essentially formed by the right ventricle and to a lesser extent by the left ventricle. The border between the ventricles is characterised on the outer surface by the Sulcus interventricularis anterior. The **R. interventricularis anterior (4)** from the A. coronaria sinistra runs in this sulcus.

From the right ventricle, the **Truncus pulmonalis (5)** ascends to the left. It splits into the **A. pulmonalis dextra (6a)** and the **A. pulmonalis sinistra (6b)**, which already lie outside the pericardium.

The **Aorta ascendens (7)** here leaves the left ventricle, which is mostly hidden in this view. It continues into the **Arcus aortae (aortic arch, 8)** outside of the pericardium. The **Truncus brachiocephalicus (9)**, the **A. carotis communis sinistra (10)** and the **A. subclavia sinistra (11)**, which supply the upper extremities and the head, arise from the aortic arch.

The **Lig. arteriosum (12)** spans the Arcus aortae and the Truncus pulmonalis. It is a vestige of the Ductus arteriosus [Botalli], which forms a connection between the pulmonary and the systemic circulation in fetal circulation.

The Sulcus coronarius forms the border between the ventricles and the atria. Amongst others, the **A. coronaria dextra (13)** runs in it, as well as the **V. cardiaca parva (14)**.

The **right atrium (Atrium dextrum, 15)** forms the right side of the heart and ventrally encompasses the Aorta ascendens with the **Auricula dextra (15a)**. The **V. cava superior (upper caval vein, 16)** flows cranially into the right atrium. In this view, from the left atrium (Atrium sinistrum) only the **Auricula sinistra (17a)** is visible, extending to the ventral surface between the left ventricle and the Truncus pulmonalis.

Dorsal view   In the dorsal view, the **Facies diaphragmatica (18)** of the heart is visible. For the most part it is formed by the left ventricle and to a lesser extent by the right ventricle.

The border between the ventricles is represented by the Sulcus interventricularis posterior, in which the **R. interventricularis posterior (19)** runs, provided by the A. coronaria dextra. On the border between the ventricles and the atriums, the **R. circumflexus (20)** from the A. coronaria sinistra and the **Sinus coronarius (21)** runs in the Sulcus coronarius. The Sinus coronarius is provided by the V. cardiaca magna and carries a majority of the venal blood of the heart to the right atrium.

The space of the dorsal side of the heart is almost completely filled by the **left atrium (Atrium sinistrum, 17)**. Blood mainly from four **Vv. pulmonales (22)** flows into the left atrium.

On the right side of the heart, a small part of the **right atrium (15)** is visible. **V. cava superior enters cranially (16),** and the **V. cava inferior enters caudally (23)**.

Clinical remarks

A simple examination to determine the size and shape of the heart uses a thoracic X-ray image in the **posterior-anterior (sagittal) beam path.** Therefore it is important to know the structures which form the marginal contours of the heart on the X-ray image. On the right side of the heart these are in craniocaudal order: the V. cava superior and the right atrium, on the left side of the heart: the Arcus aortae, the Truncus pulmonalis, the left auricle and the left ventricle.

The right ventricle and the left atrium can be assessed with an X-ray image of the thorax in the **transverse beam path**.

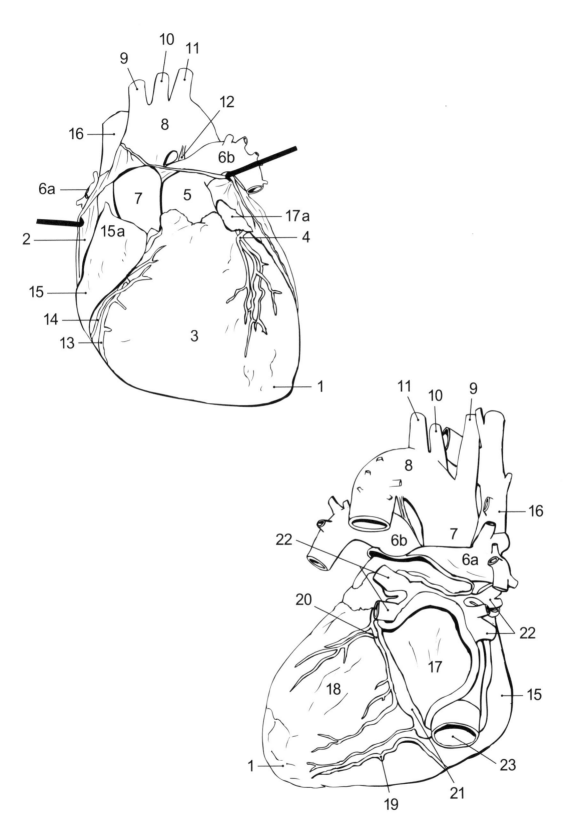

Abb. 4.2

73

4.3 Chambers of the heart

Right atrium and right ventricle A textured and a smooth-walled part can be recognized on the inner walls of the **right atrium**.

The **textured part** corresponds to the **right auricle (1)** and is defined by the **Mm. pectinati (2)**. The Mm. pectinati protrude like the teeth of a comb into the lumen of the right atrium. The right auricle represents the developmentally older part of the right atrium.

The **smooth-walled part (3)** only becomes part of the right atrium later on. It is formed by the tissue of the **Sinus venosus**, which during development connects the two caval veins.

Into the right atrium flow

- cranially, the **V. cava superior (4)**
- caudally, the **V. cava inferior (5)**

The blood flow from the V. cava inferior is guided through a valve, the **Valvula venae cavae inferioris (6)**, onto the former Foramen ovale. In this short circuit between the right and left atrium, extant from fetal blood circulation, another indentation in the adult heart, the **Fossa ovalis (7)**, can be discerned. It has a prominent oval margin, the **Limbus fossae ovalis (8)**. In the fetal circulation, the Valvula venae cavae inferioris guides the oxygen-rich blood from the lower caval vein via the Foramen ovale into the left atrium and thereby bypasses the circulation of the lungs.

In the right atrium, the mouth or orifice of the **Sinus coronarius (9)**, can be seen, into which flows most of the venal blood of the heart.

At the border of the **right ventricle** is the **Valva atrioventricularis dextra (tricuspid valve = Valva tricuspidalis, 10a–c)**. The tricuspid valve consists of three cusps:

- **Cuspis anterior (anterior cusp, 10a)**
- **Cuspis posterior (posterior cusp, 10b)**
- **Cuspis septalis (septal cusp, 10c)**

Inserting at the cusps, with thin tendinous cords, are the **Chordae tendineae (11):**

- **M. papillaris anterior (anterior papillary muscle, 12a)**
- **M. papillaris posterior (posterior papillary muscle, 12b)**
- **M. papillaris septalis (septal papillary muscle, 12c)**

The septal papillary muscle is often only sparsely formed. With a ventricle systole, the papillary muscles prevent the cusps from everting in the right atrium and thereby ensure the tight closure of the tricuspid valve. In the ventricle lumen, the mesh-like muscular columns of the **Trabeculae carneae** are visible.

Left ventricle The inner walls of the left ventricle also consist of Trabeculae carneae. Because of the predominant pressure ratio, the wall of the left ventricle is visibly thicker than that of the right ventricle.

The **Valva atrioventricularis sinistra (mitral valve = Valva mitralis, 13a and b)** is on the border between the left atrium and the left ventricle. The mitral valve consists of two cusps:

- the **Cuspis anterior (anterior cusp, 13a)**
- the **Cuspis posterior (posterior cusp, 13b)**

The **M. papillaris anterior (anterior papillary muscle, 14a)** and the **M. papillaris posterior (posterior papillary muscle, 14b)** insert on this atrioventricular valve via the **Chordae tendineae (11)**.

In the area of the outflow tract, the left ventricle is closed with a **semilunar valve (Valva aortae = aortic valve, 15a–c)** through to the **Aorta ascendens (16)**. This valve consists of:

- **Valvula semilunaris sinistra (15a)**
- **Valvula semilunaris posterior (15b)**
- **Valvula semilunaris dextra (15c)**

The outflow tracts of the right and left coronary artery (Aa. coronariae dextra und sinistra) are visible above the Valvulae semilunares dextra and sinistra.

Note

There are four valves in the heart, acting as valves between the chambers of the heart. They consist of endocardial duplicatures and open and close passively due to differences in pressure between the atria and the chambers and/or the chambers and the arteries near the heart.

Valve	Type	Position	Property/Characteristic
Tricuspid valve	atrioventricular valve	right atrium → right ventricle	3 leaflets or cusps (anterior, posterior, septal)
Pulmonary valve	semilunar valve	right ventricle → Truncus pulmonalis	3 pocket-shaped leaflets or cusps (left, right, anterior)
Bicuspid valve	atrioventricular valve	left atrium → left ventricle	2 leaflets or cusps (anterior, posterior)
Aortic valve	semilunar valve	left ventricle → Aorta ascendens	3 pocket-shaped leaflets or cusps (left, right, posterior)

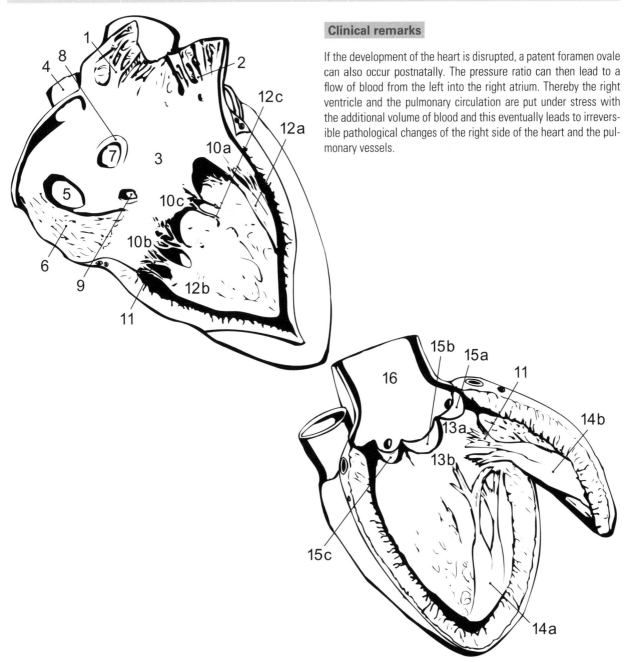

Clinical remarks

If the development of the heart is disrupted, a patent foramen ovale can also occur postnatally. The pressure ratio can then lead to a flow of blood from the left into the right atrium. Thereby the right ventricle and the pulmonary circulation are put under stress with the additional volume of blood and this eventually leads to irreversible pathological changes of the right side of the heart and the pulmonary vessels.

Abb. 4.3

4.4 Coronary arteries

The heart is supplied with blood via the **Aa. coronariae dextra (1)** and **sinistra (2)** (coronary vessels). Both arteries originate from the Aorta ascendens. They arise from immediately above the **Valvulae semilunares dextra (3)** and **sinistra (4)** of the aortic valve.

A. coronaria dextra   The **A. coronaria dextra (right coronary artery, 1)** runs in an arch along the border between the right atrium and the right ventricle in the **Sulcus coronarius** to the Facies diaphragmatica of the heart. It provides the **R. ventricularis dexter (1a)** and the **R. marginalis dexter (1b)** to the right ventricle. Additionally, it supplies large areas of the right atrium via the **Rr. atriales (1c)**. On the Facies diaphragmatica it turns around from the Sulcus coronarius into the **Sulcus interventricularis posterior** and ends here as the **R. interventricularis posterior (1d)**. The R. interventricularis posterior supplies the right ventricle on the Facies diaphragmatica, parts of the left ventricle and the posterior parts of the ventricular septum via the Rr. septales posteriores.

A. coronaria sinistra   The **A. coronaria sinistra (left coronary artery, 2)** forms a short stem, situated between the left auricle and the Truncus pulmonalis. Shortly thereafter, the stem bifurcates into:

- the **R. interventricularis anterior (2a)**. It runs in the **anterior longitudinal** sulcus in the direction of the Apex cordis and supplies small parts of the right ventricle, those parts of the left ventricle in the region of the Facies sternocostalis, and via the Rr. septales anteriores, the majority of the ventricular septum.
- the **R. circumflexus (2b)**. It runs in the Sulcus coronaries in an arch to the Facies diaphragmatica and, along its course, provides branches to the left atrium (not shown). Via the **R. marginalis sinister (2c)** and the **R. posterior ventriculi sinistri (2d)** , it supplies the left ventricle.

Note

The strength as well as the branching pattern of the coronary arteries are variable. The supply of the Facies diaphragmatica and of the ventricular septum can preferentially take place from the right or the left coronary arteries. Depending on the supply area, a balanced blood supply, or a dominant right or left blood supply are differentiated.

Clinical remarks

The coronary arteries show the smallest anastomoses, but from a functional perspective they need to be seen as terminal arteries. Complete or partial closures of coronary artery branches cannot be compensated for via other branches. This results in a decreased blood flow or necrosis of the muscle of the heart. Clinically this presents as **angina-pectoris** or as a **myocardial infarction**.

If the A. coronaria dextra, the R. interventricularis anterior and the R. circumflexus are constricted at the same time, it is known as a **triple vessel disease**. A **posterior myocardial infarction** indicates infarctions in the anatomical Facies diaphragmatica area.

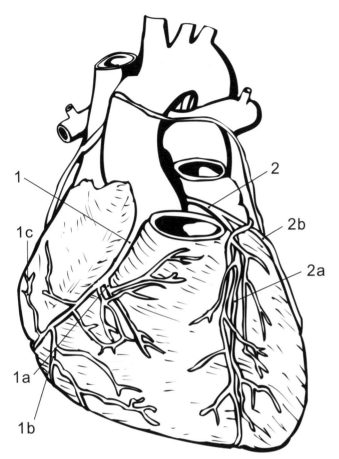

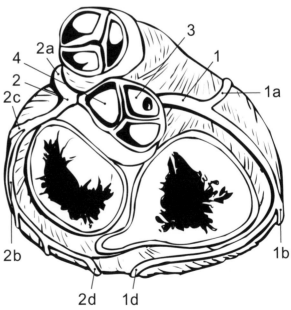

Abb. 4.4

4.5 Lungs

Both of the lungs (**Pulmones dexter and sinister**) are covered by the **Pleura visceralis** and more or less fill the respective breathing-dependent **pleural cavities**. The size and the shape of the lungs adapt to the pleural cavities and the adjacent organs, so that the dissected lungs show imprints of the adjacent structures.

Right lung The right lung (Pulmo dexter, illustration above) consists of three lobes:
- the **upper lobe (Lobus superior, Ia)**
- the **middle lobe (Lobus medius, II)**
- the **lower lobe (Lobus inferior, IIIa)**

The pulmonary lobes are separated from each other by fissures, which extend almost to the **hilum of the lung (IVa)**. The fissures enable the lobes to slide against each other during breathing. The **Fissura obliqua (1a)** divides the lower lobes from the other two lobes. The **Fissura horizontalis (2)** divides the upper from the middle lobe.

Besides the lobular division, three surfaces can be differentiated on the lungs:
- the **Facies costalis (3a)**, which faces the ribs
- the **Facies mediastinalis (4a)**, which borders the mediastinum
- the **Facies diaphragmatica (5a)**, which abuts the diaphragm

The **upper lobe (Ia)** forms the rounded-off **apex of the lung (Apex pulmonis, 6a)**, which is positioned in situ in the Fossa supraclavicularis major. The **middle lobe (IIa)** essentially faces ventrally, while the **lower lobe (IIIa)** abuts the diaphragm and the dorsal sections of the ribs.

In the area of the **hilum of the lung (IVa)**, the vessels of the lung and the primary bronchus enter the lungs and form the **roots of the lung (Radix pulmonis)**.

The **right primary bronchus (Bronchus principalis dexter, 7)** is situated furthest dorsally in the right hilum of the lung. The **A. pulmonalis dextra (8)**, which has already been divided into its branches in the illustration, is ventral of the primary bronchus and is situated at the same level. The **Vv. pulmonales dextrae (9)** lie below the artery and obliquely anterior, caudal of the primary bronchus. The hilum of the lung is lined by the **pleural cuff (10a)** of the parietal pleura, which here passes into the visceral pleura. Caudally of the hilum structure, this cuff continues and forms the **Lig. pulmonale (11a)**.

Left lung The left lung (Pulmo sinister, illustration below) consists of only two lobes:
- an **upper lobe (Lobus superior, Ib)**
- a **lower lobe (Lobus inferior, IIIb)**

There is no middle lobe. Upper and lower lobes are divided from each other by the **Fissura obliqua (1b)**. The left lung also shows a **Facies costalis (3b)**, a **Facies mediastinalis (4b)** and a **Facies diaphragmatica (5b)**.

The **upper lobe** forms the **apex of the lung (Apex pulmonis, 6b) , 6a)**, and large parts abut the mediastinum and the ventral sections of the ribs. The Facies mediastinalis is compressed by the heart to a deep **Impressio cardiaca (12)**, whereby a tongue-shaped projection develops, the **Lingula pulmonis (13)**, at the caudal end of the upper lobe.

The **lower lobe** abuts the diaphragm and borders the dorsal sections of the ribs. The **hilum structures (IVb)** are arranged differently in the left lung than in the right: the **left primary bronchus (Bronchus principalis sinister, 14)** lies furthest dorsally but below the **A. pulmonalis sinistra (15)**. The **left veins of the lung (Vv. pulmonales sinistrae, 16)** are situated at the front and below the primary bronchus. The left hilum of the lung encompasses the **pleural cuff (10b)** of the parietal and visceral pleura, which continues into the **Lig. pulmonale (11b)**.

Note

Right lung	Upper, middle, lower lobe	In the hilum, the primary bronchus and the A. pulmonalis are on the same level.
Left lung	Upper, lower lobe	The A. pulmonalis lies in the hilum, cranially of the primary bronchus.

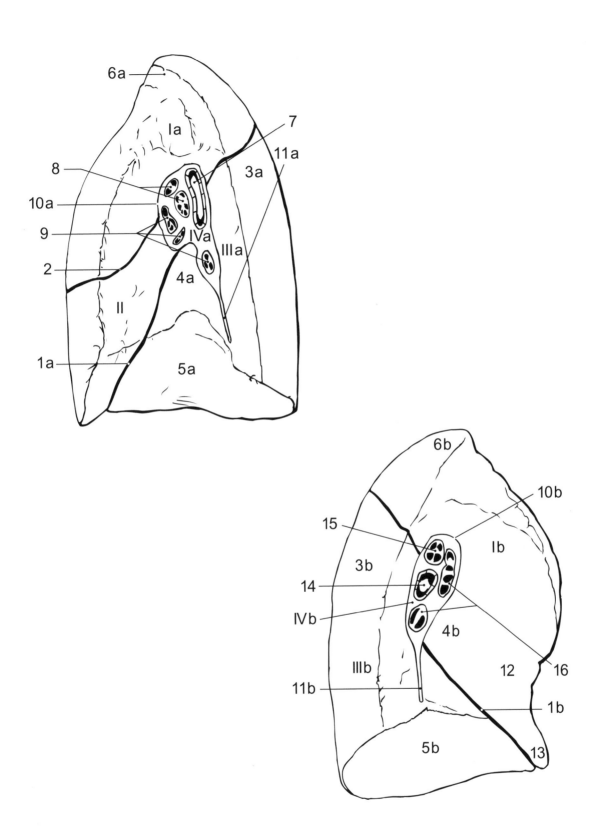

Abb. 4.5

79

4.6 Mediastinum, view from the right

The mediastinum becomes visible from the right by removing the ribs on the right side, the parietal pleura and the right lung. The dome-shaped, arched **diaphragm (Diaphragma, 1)** borders the thoracic cavity caudally. The **Thymus (2)** and the **pericardium (3)**, can both be seen at the front of the mediastinum, bordering the sternum and the ventral ribs.

Hilum of the lung   After removal of the lung, the structures of the **right hilum of the lung (4)** become visible:
* the right **primary bronchus (Bronchus principalis dexter, 5)**
* the **A. pulmonalis dextra (6)**, which lies at the same level
* caudally thereof, the **Vv. pulmonales dextrae (7)**

Caudally of the hilum, the pleural cuff continues as the **Lig. pulmonale (8)**.

N. phrenicus, N. vagus and Truncus sympathicus   The **N. phrenicus (9)** runs ventrally of the hilum of the lung. It originates from the Plexus cervicalis, descends in the thorax and innervates the pericardium, the mediastinal Pleura parietalis and the diaphragm.

The **N. vagus (N. X, 10)** runs dorsally of the hilum of the lung. It provides the **N. laryngeus recurrens (11)** to the larynx shortly after entering the upper thoracic aperture. Descending further, it attaches in the posterior mediastinum to the **oesophagus (12)** and forms a plexus here with the N. vagus of the other side. Together with the oesophagus, it eventually passes through the diaphragm into the abdominal cavity. Along this pathway, the N. vagus provides numerous small branches for the parasympathetic innervation of the thoracic viscera.

Further dorsally, the **Truncus sympathicus (sympathetic trunk, 13)** runs paravertebrally. Its ganglia provide nerve fibres to the peripheral nerves, e.g. the **intercostal nerves (Nn. intercostales, 14)**, and for the sympathetic innervation of the thoracic organs. The **N. splanchnicus major (15)** and the **N. splanchnicus minor (16)** have already exited before it passes through the diaphragm. Separated from the sympathetic trunk, they both pass through the diaphragm and run in the prevertebral ganglia which innervate the abdominal organs.

V. azygos   In the posterior mediastinum, the **V. azygos (17)** runs on the right side. Amongst others, it incorporates tributaries from the **intercostal veins (Vv. intercostales, 18)** and, cranially of the hilum of the lung, it turns to ventral. Eventually it flows into the **V. cava superior (19)** near the heart.

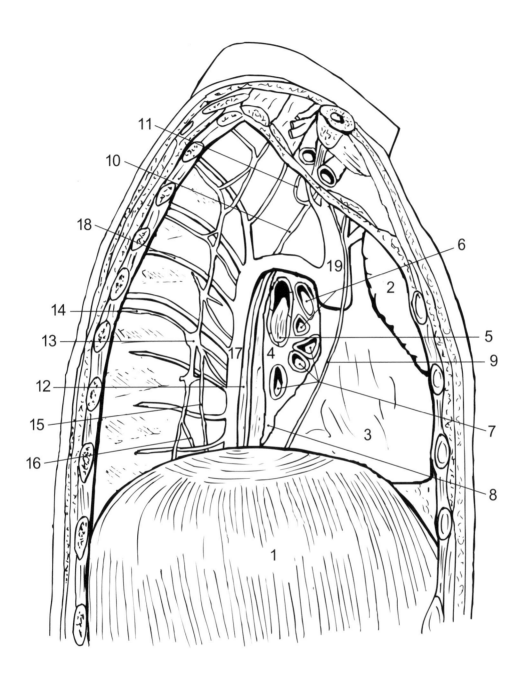

Abb. 4.6

81

4.7 Mediastinum, view from the left

The mediastinum becomes visible by removing the ribs, the left lung and the parietal pleura. The dome-shaped, arched **diaphragm (Diaphragma, 1)** borders the thoracic cavity caudally. The **thymus (2)** and the **pericardium (3)** can both be seen in the anterior mediastinum, bordering the sternum and the ventral ribs.

Hilum of the lung
After removal of the lung, the structures of the **left hilum of the lung** are visible:
- the left **primary bronchus (Bronchus principalis sinister, 4)**
- the **A. pulmonalis sinistra (5)**, which lies further cranially, as well as
- ventrally and caudally of the primary bronchus, the **Vv. pulmonales sinistrae (6)**

N. phrenicus, N. vagus and Truncus sympathicus
The **N. phrenicus (7)** runs ventrally of the hilum of the lung. It originates from the Plexus cervicalis, descends in the thorax and innervates the pericardium, the mediastinal Pleura parietalis and the diaphragm.

The **N. vagus (N. X, 8)** runs dorsally of the hilum of the lung. On its downward path, it attaches to the **oesophagus (9)** in the posterior mediastinum and forms a plexus here with the N. vagus of the other side. Together with the oesophagus, it eventually passes through the diaphragm into the abdominal cavity. Along this pathway, the N. vagus provides numerous small branches for the parasympathetic innervation of the thoracic viscera.

Further dorsally, the **Truncus sympathicus (sympathetic trunk, 10)** runs paravertebrally. Its ganglia provide nerve fibres to the peripheral nerves, e.g. the **intercostal nerves (Nn. intercostales, 11)**, and for the sympathetic innervation of the thoracic organs. The **N. splanchnicus major (12)** and the **N. splanchnicus minor (13)** have already exited before it passes through the diaphragm. Separated from the sympathetic trunk, they both pass through the diaphragm and run in the prevertebral ganglia which innervate the abdominal organs.

Aorta thoracica
The **Arcus aortae (aortic arch, 14a)** runs from the right and from ventral to the left and dorsally. Thereby it ends up immediately cranial of the left hilum of the lung and then continues as the **Aorta descendens (14b)** in the posterior mediastinum. The **A. carotis communis sinistra (15)** and the **A. subclavia sinistra (16)** also exit in the aortic arch. The **intercostal arteries (Aa. intercostales, e.g. 17)** originate from the Aorta descendens. Descending in the posterior mediastinum, the Aorta descendens eventually passes through its own opening in the diaphragm.

V. hemiazygos
In the posterior mediastinum, the **V. hemiazygos (18)** runs along the left side. Amongst others, it receives tributaries from the intercostal veins and turns at the level of the 7th–10th thoracic vertebrae behind the Aorta descendens to the right. Here it continues cranially in the **V. hemiazygos accessoria (19)**. It collects the blood from the upper intercostal spaces and flows into the V. brachiocephalica sinistra or shows a direct connection to the **V. cava superior (20)**. The V. hemiazygos flows in the posterior mediastinum into the V. azygos.

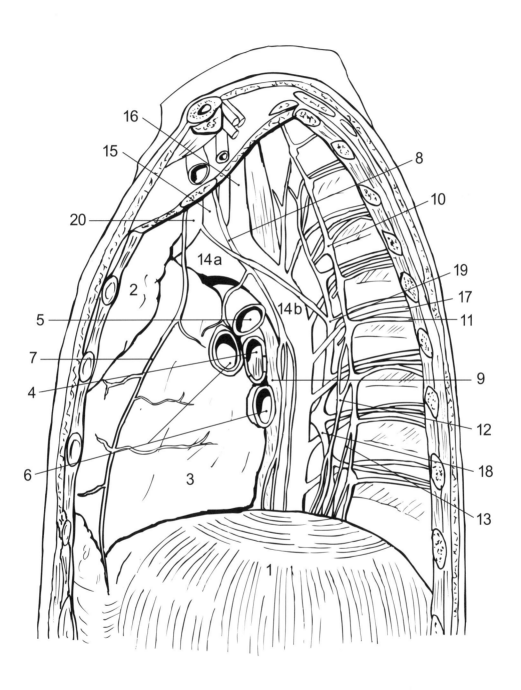

Abb. 4.7

4.8 Posterior mediastinum, view from ventral I

The structures of the upper and the posterior lower mediastinum become visible after removing the ribs, sternum, thymus, lungs, heart and the serous membranes.

Trachea   Coming from the Spatium viscerale of the neck, the **trachea (1)** passes into the upper thoracic outlet. Its tracheal bifurcation, the **Bifurcatio tracheae (2)**, lies at the level of the 4th thoracic vertebrae. The **Bronchi principales dexter and sinister (right and left primary bronchus, 3a and b)** leave from the trachea. The right primary bronchus has a slightly larger lumen than the left and descends less sharply from the trachea to lateral.

Oesophagus   Initially hidden by the trachea, the **Oesophagus (4)** becomes visible underneath the Bifurcatio tracheae. In this area, it abuts the posterior wall of the pericardium and is therefore directly adjacent to the left atrium. In conjunction with the oesophagus, both **Nn. vagi (N. X, 5a and b)** run in the posterior lower mediastinum.

Just after their entry into the upper thoracic outlet, the Nn. vagi provide the Nn. laryngei recurrentes to the larynx. The right **N. laryngeus recurrens (6a)** hereby loops around the **A. subclavia dextra (7),** here partially removed, while the left **N. laryngeus recurrens (6b)** turns back around the **aortic arch (8a)** in a cranial direction. Both the Nn. vagi exchange fibres with each other and thereby form the **Plexus oesophageus (9)** on the oesophagus. The oesophagus and the Nn. vagi pass through the **diaphragm (Diaphragma, 10)** via the **Hiatus oesophageus**. Immediately below the diaphragm, the Nn. vagi provide **branches (Rr. gastrici anteriores, 5c)** to the **stomach (11)** and then, further along the pathway, also supply most of the abdominal organs parasympathetically.

Aorta   The Aorta thoracica starts at the left ventricle with the Aorta ascendens, which here has been removed with the heart. This aortic section continues into the **Arcus aortae (aortic arch, 8a)**, from which originate the **Truncus brachiocephalicus (12)**, the **A. carotis communis sinistra (13)** and the **A. subclavia sinistra (14)**. The aortic arch then turns caudally and thereby ends up cranially of the **left primary bronchus (3b)**. As a continuation of the aortic arch, the **Aorta descendens (8b)** runs slightly to the left of the midline, descending in the posterior lower mediastinum. It passes through the diaphragm in the area of the Hiatus aorticus.

Truncus sympathicus   The **Truncus sympathicus (sympathetic trunk, 15a and b)** runs paravertebrally on both sides. Along its pathway, it provides fibres to peripheral nerves, such as the **intercostal nerves (16)**, and for the sympathetic innervation of the thoracic organs.

Clinical remarks

The oesophagus is underneath the Bifurcatio tracheae at the back of the heart, and thereby abuts the left atrium. To gauge the size of the left atrium, a **thoracic X-ray with a transverse projection** is needed with an orally administered X-ray contrast agent (barium meal). If filling the oesophagus with the contrast agent displaces it, this is an indication of a pathological enlargement of the left atrium. In addition, a sonographic depiction of the heart is possible with an ultrasonic probe introduced via the oesophagus.

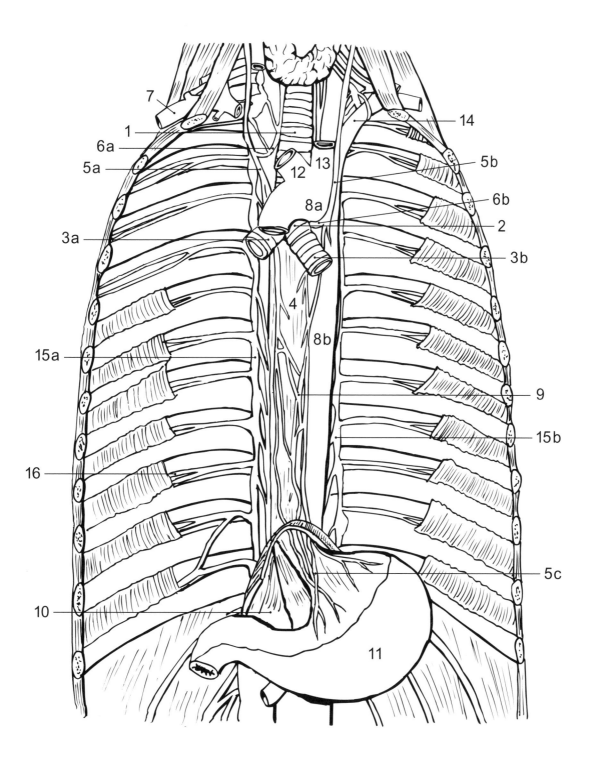

Abb. 4.8

85

4.9 Posterior mediastinum, view from ventral II

The furthest dorsally situated structures of the posterior lower mediastinum become visible with resection of the middle and distal **oesophagus (1)**.

Ductus thoracicus The **Ductus thoracicus (thoracic duct, 3)** becomes visible between the **Aorta descendens (2)** and the spinal column. The Ductus thoracicus is a large lymph vessel with valves. It originates from the Cisterna chyli (not shown) immediately below the **diaphragm (Diaphragma, 4)** and drains the lymph of the lower half of the body and the abdominal organs to the left venous angle between the V. subclavia sinistra and the V. jugularis interna sinistra. It was given its German name of 'milk breast duct' due to the milky color caused by the dietary fats transported in the lymph after a meal. Situated as it is between the Aorta descendens and the spinal column, it leads to the Ductus thoracicus being compressed by pulse waves running across the aorta. Additionally, the valve system in the Ductus thoracicus supports the lymph flow to cranial.

V. azygos, V. hemiazygos The **V. azygos (5)** is visible slightly to the right from the midline. It collects the venous blood from the right intercostal spaces and runs in an arch via the **right primary bronchus (6)** to the V. cava superior. At the level of the 7th–10th thoracic vertebrae, the **V. hemiazygos (7)** flows from the left into the V. azygos.

Truncus sympathicus The **Truncus sympathicus (8)** is visible on the right side. It provides the **N. splanchnicus major (9)** from the 6th–9th thoracic ganglia and the **N. splanchnicus minor (10)** from the 10th–11th thoracic ganglia to medial. The Nn. splanchnici follow a descending path, mostly via the medial part of the diaphragm into the abdominal cavity. There they end in the prevertebral sympathetic ganglia, which innervate the abdominal organs sympathetically.

Removal of the stomach makes it possible to see the opening, the **Hiatus aorticus (11)**, through which the **Aorta descendens (2)** passes into the abdominal cavity via the diaphragm.

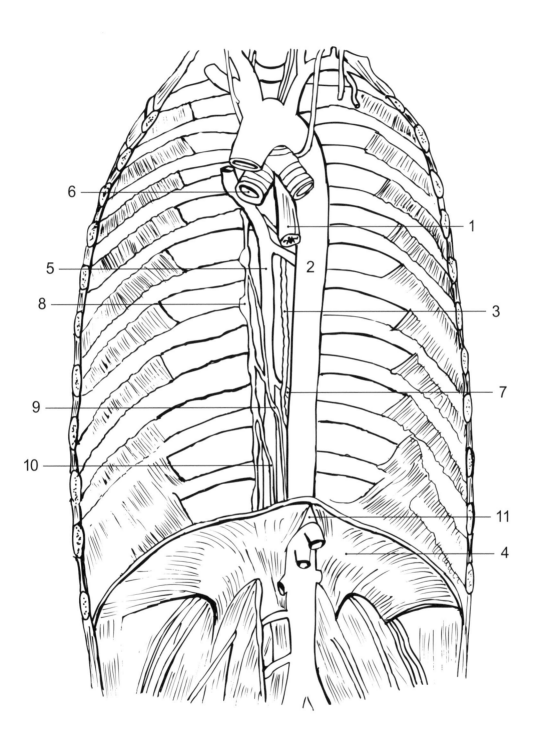

6

1

5

2

8

3

9

7

10

11

4

Abb. 4.9

87

4.10 Diaphragm, caudal view

The diaphragm (Diaphragma) is the most important muscle for breathing and is innervated by the N. phrenicus. As a dome-shaped sheet of muscle, it divides the thorax from the abdominal cavity. Due to the origin of the diaphragm, there are three parts:

- **Pars lumbalis (1a–d)**
- **Pars costalis (2)**
- **Pars sternalis (3)**

The three parts merge at the highest point of the diaphragmatic dome in the fascial **Centrum tendineum (4)**. In the diaphragm there are openings for structures to pass from the thorax into the abdominal cavity and back again.

Pars lumbalis The **Pars lumbalis (1a–d)** originates from the lumbar spine and two fascial arches:

- from the **Lig. arcuatum mediale (5a and b)**, which spans the **M. psoas (6a and b)** (psoas arcade)
- from the **Lig. arcuatum laterale (7a and b)**, which straddles the **M. quadratus lumborum (8a and b)** (quadratus arcade)

On each side one can respectively see a **Crus mediale (1a and b)** and a **Crus laterale (1c and d)**. The **Crura medialia** originates from the lumbar spine. The Crus mediale on the left mostly originates at a deeper point than on the right. The **Crura lateralia** originates from the above mentioned tendinous arches. Between the Crura mediale and laterale, the **Truncus sympathicus** (not shown) passes through the diaphragm on both sides. The V. azygos runs on the right and the V. hemiazygos on the left through the Crus mediale as well as on both sides of the Nn. splanchnici. The medial muscle fibres of both the Crura medialia run cranially into the **Lig. arcuatum medianum (9)**, which encircle the **Hiatus aorticus (10)** the opening for the aorta and the Ductus thoracicus. The opening for the oesophagus and the Nn. vagi, the **Hiatus oesophageus (11)**, lies ventrally.

Pars costalis The **Pars costalis (2)** originates from the caudal six ribs. Between the Pars lumbalis and the Pars costalis there is on both sides a space devoid of muscle, the **Trigonum lumbocostale (12a and b)**.

Pars sternalis The **Pars sternalis (3)** originates from the back of the sternum and the posterior sheet of the rectal sheath. Between the Pars sternalis and the Pars costalis a small gap devoid of muscle remains on both sides, **Trigonum sternocostale** **(cleft of Larrey, 13a and b)**, through which the A. and V. thoracica interna respectively run from the thorax into the rectal sheath.

Centrum tendineum The tendinous sheet of the **Centrum tendineum (4)** connects the muscle fibres of the various diaphragmatic sections with each other. Cranially the pericardium lies on the Centrum tendineum, leading to shifting of the heart depending on respiration. In the right part of the Centrum tendineum there is an opening, the **Foramen venae cavae (14)**, for the lower caval vein to pass through.

Clinical remarks

Abdominal viscera can herniate into the thoracic space through the openings of the diaphragm and through its areas devoid of muscles. **Hernias** mostly occur in the area of the **Hiatus oesophageus** (hiatus hernias) and in the **Trigonum lumbocostale** (Bochdalek triangle).

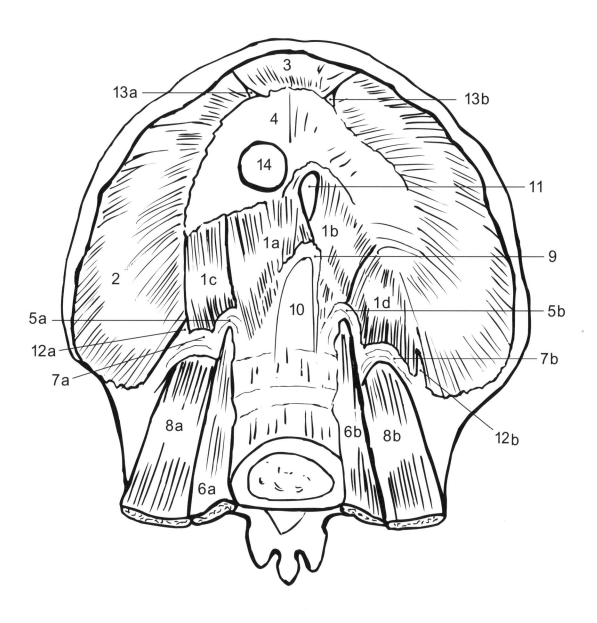

Abb. 4.10

89

5.1 Abdominal muscles

The muscles of the abdomen extend from the lower edge of the thorax up to the upper edge of the pelvis. They run straight as well as obliquely. This muscle layer enables the abdominal muscles to **rotate and bend the torso over and to the side**. Besides enabling the spinal column to move in different ways, tensing the abdominal muscles increases **intra abdominal pressure**, which pushes the diaphragm cranially if the glottis is opened and thereby induces a forced exhalation (cough). With the glottis closed, the diaphragm cannot expand cranially, and thereby the increased intraabdominal pressure interacts with the abdominal organs. This function of the abdominal muscles is significant during micturition, defecation and when supporting labour while giving birth.

The abdominal muscles are innervated by caudal intercostal nerves and by the Nn. iliohypogastricus and ilioinguinalis from the Plexus lumbalis.

The anterior wall of the abdomen contains four muscles:
- **M. rectus abdominis (1)**
- **M. obliquus externus abdominis (2)**
- **M. obliquus internus abdominis (3)**
- **M. transversus abdominis**

M. rectus abdominis Both of the **Mm. recti abdominis (1)** run straight down caudally from the Proc. xiphoideus and the cartilage of the 5th–7th ribs to the cranial edge of the Os pubis and the symphysis. The Mm. recti abdominis lie in a quiver-shaped sheath, the **rectus sheath (Vagina musculi recti abdominis)**, which is formed by the aponeurosis of the lateral oblique and straight abdominal muscles and by the Fascia transversalis (➤ Chap. 5.2). In the diagram, the right side of the ventral membrane of the **rectus sheath (1a)** has been opened, so that the M. rectus abdominis is now visible. The M. rectus abdominis is subdivided by 3–4 **Intersectiones tendineae (1b)** into muscle bellies. The Intersectiones tendineae are fused with the ventral membrane of the rectus sheath and enable a progressive contraction of the muscles.

The Mm. recti abdominis enable the torso to bend forwards and to interact with abdominal pressure.

M. obliquus externus abdominis The **M. obliquus externus abdominis (2)** runs from above and posterior, in an oblique line inferiorly and anteriorly. It originates from the 6th–12th ribs, where its fleshy digitations receive the corresponding processes of the **M. serratus anterior (4)** and the M. latissimus dorsi (not shown). The upper digitations pass over the edge of the M. rectus abdominis into an aponeurosis, together forming the **rectus sheath (1a)**. The lower digitations proceed to the ventral section of the Crista iliaca up to the Spina iliaca anterior superior.

The M. obliquus externus abdominis is involved with intra-abdominal pressure as well as with the rotation and forwards/side-bending of the torso.

M. obliquus internus abdominis The **M. obliquus internus abdominis (3)** can be seen in the depiction on the left side of the torso, after the digitations of the **M. obliquus externus abdominis (2a)** have been severed and folded back medially. The fibres of the M. obliquus internus abdominis run almost vertically to those of the M. obliquus externus abdominis. They originate dorsally from the Fascia thoracolumbalis and from the Crista iliaca up to the inguinal ligament. The cranial sections ascend obliquely to the caudal ribs. The middle and lower sections pass over into an **aponeurosis (3a)**, which form a part of the rectus sheath. The caudal sections of the M. obliquus internus abdominis run horizontally, or even obliquely descending.

The M. obliquus internus abdominis is involved with intra-abdominal pressure as well as with the roation and forward/side-bending of the torso.

The **M. cremaster (5)** branches off from the lowest fibres of the M. obliquus internus abdominis. It runs in the spermatic cord via the inguinal canal to the testicles (➤ Chap. 5.3).

M. transversus abdominis The M. transversus abdominis lies below the M. obliquus internus abdominis and is therefore not visible here. Its fibres run horizontally. It originates at the caudal ribs, and the Fascia thoracolumbalis at the Procc. costales of the lumbar vertebra and the Crista iliaca. Medially it passes over into an aponeurosis, which is involved in the formation of the rectus sheath.

The M. transversus abdominis is involved with intra-abdominal pressure.

Clinical remarks

Great care should be taken not to injure the structure of the abdominal muscles, avoiding for instance later **incisional hernias** during surgical procedures in the abdomen.

During an **appendicitis** operation, the Mm. obliqui externus abdominis and internus abdominis, as well as transversus abdominis, should therefore each be divided following the direction of their fibres **(McBurney's incision)**.

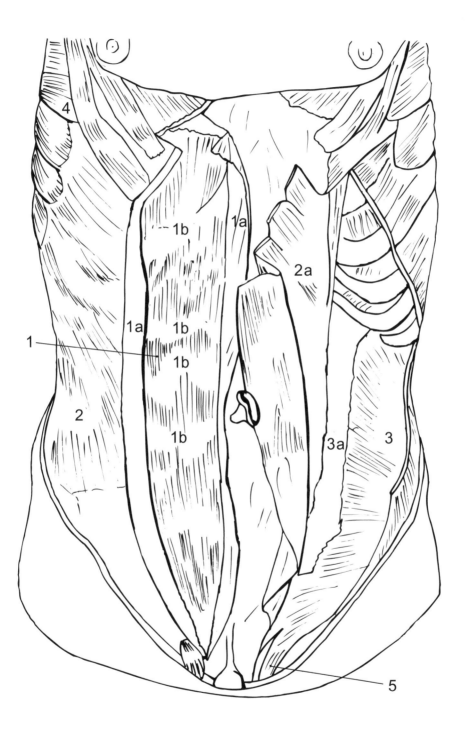

Abb. 5.1

5.2 Rectus sheath

The **M. rectus abdominis (1a–c)** is the direct antagonist of the **M. erector spinae (2)** . Both the Mm. recti abdominis respectively lie in a quiver-shaped sheath (**Rectus sheath = Vagina musculi recti abdominis**), formed by the aponeurosis of the lateral stomach muscles (M. obliquus externus abdominis, M. obliquus internus abdominis, M. transversus abdominis) and the Fascia transversalis. The structure of the rectus sheath is, however, not the same in all the sections, as it varies in a craniocaudal direction. The rectus sheath consists of a ventral and a dorsal membrane.

Cranial section of the rectus sheath (A) The cranial part of the rectus sheath lies between the costal arches. Here the ventral membrane is only formed by the **aponeurosis (3a)** of the **M. obliquus externus abdominis (4a)** and is relatively thin. The dorsal membrane of the rectus sheath consists here of muscle fibres of the **M. transversus abdominis (5a)** and the **Fascia transversalis (6a)**.

Middle section of the rectus sheath (B) The middle section of the rectus sheath is shown here at the level of the navel. The ventral membrane is formed by the **aponeurosis (3b)** of the **M. obliquus externus abdominis (4b)** and by half of the **aponeurosis (7b)** of the **M. obliquus internus abdominis (8b)**. The other half of the **internal aponeurosis (7b)**, the **aponeurosis (9b)** of the **M. transversus abdominis (5b)** and the **Fascia transversalis (6b),** form the dorsal membrane.

Caudal section of the rectus sheath (C) The caudal section of the rectus sheath lies below the navel. Here the aponeurosis of the **M. obliquus externus abdominis (3c)**, **M. obliquus internus abdominis (8c)** and the **M. transversus abdominis (5c)** run entirely in front of the **M. rectus abdominis (1c)** and form the ventral membrane of the rectus sheath. The dorsal membrane here consists exclusively of the **Fascia transversalis (6c)**.

In the area of transition from the middle into the caudal section of the rectus sheath, the dorsal membrane becomes noticeably thinner. Studying this area on a dissection, behind the M. rectus abdominis, the transition known as the **Linea arcuata** becomes visible.

In the midline, the aponeuroses of the lateral stomach muscles interlock with each other, thereby forming the **Linea alba (9a–c)**. This line is thin and wide above the navel but thick and narrow below.

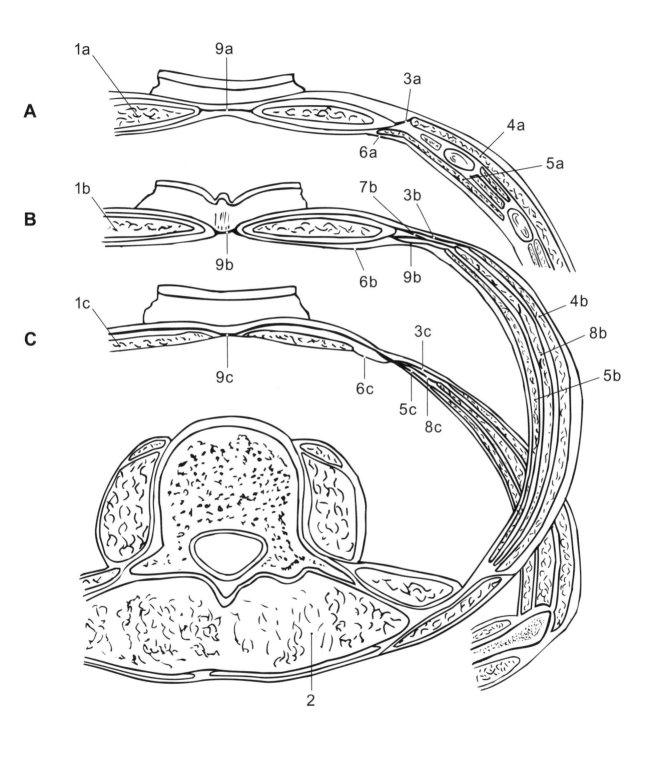

Abb. 5.2

5.3 Inguinal canal

Boundaries of the inguinal canal   The **inguinal canal (Canalis inguinalis)** passes through the wall of the abdomen from the **Anulus inguinalis profundus (1)** to the **Anulus inguinalis superficialis (2)**. Thereby it runs from cranial and lateral to caudal and medial through the wall of the abdomen. The inguinal canal is approx. 4–5 cm long and consists of two narrow and two wide boundaries:

* The roof of the inguinal canal is formed by the lower margin of the **M. obliquus internus abdominis (3)** and the **M. transversus abdominis**.
* The floor is represented by the **Lig. inguinale (inguinal ligament, 4)**.
* The aponeurosis of the **M. obliquus externus abdominis (5)** forms the front wall.
* The back wall consists of the **Fascia transversalis (6)**. The **A.** and the **V. epigastrica inferior (7)** of the inguinal canal cross in the back wall.

The inguinal canal represents an anatomically weak spot in the wall of the abdomen (see Clinical remarks). Particular weak spots, such as the **Anuli inguinales**, are nevertheless additionally strengthened:

* The **Anulus inguinalis profundus** is covered ventrally by the caudal fibres of the M. obliquus internus abdominis.
* In the area of the **Anulus inguinalis superficialis,** the front wall is particularly thin. Here the posterior wall is particularly thickened with the **Falx inguinalis (8)**.

Scrotum and the contents of the inguinal canal   The **Descensus testis (9)** from the abdominal cavity via the inguinal canal in the scrotum causes the layers of the abdominal wall to further evert and to envelop the testes and the structures in the inguinal canal as the **Fascia spermatica externa** (formerly the **aponeurosis of the M. externus abdominis, 10**) and as the **Fascia spermatica interna** (formerly the **Fascia transversalis, 11**). The parietal peritoneum is also pouched out into the scrotum as finger-shaped **Proc. vaginalis peritonei**. The connection to the peritoneal cavity eventually closes, and vestiges of the Proc. vaginalis peritonei remain, enveloping only the testes as serous membranes, the **peri-** and **epiorchium (12)**.

The sheath and the structures within it (see table) form the **Funiculus spermaticus (spermatic cord, 13)** in men. The **Ductus deferens** (defent duct, **14**) also runs in the spermatic cord. It starts in the area of the epididymus and runs through the inguinal canal. After fusion with the excretory duct of the seminal vesicles the resulting ejaculatory duct eventually opens into the

Pars prostatica of the urethra. Because its muscle wall is thick, the Ductus deferens in the scrotum can easily be palpated as a sturdy, spherical cord.

Contents of the inguinal canal

Men	Women
• Ductus deferens (14) • A. testicularis • A. ductus deferentis • A. cremasterica • Veins (Plexus pampiniformis) • Lymph vessels • R. genitalis of the N. genitofemoralis • M. cremaster	• Lig. teres uteri • A. ligamenti teretis uteri • Veins • Lymph vessels • R. genitalis of the N. genitofemoralis

Clinical remarks

Hernias of abdominal organs can occur in the weak spots on the abdominal wall, particularly in the area of the inguinal canal. Inguinal hernias have inner hernial orifices cranial of the Lig. inguinale and are subdivided into:

* The **lateral (indirect) inguinal hernia** uses the Anulus inguinalis profundus as the inner hernial orifice. It everts out through an open Proc. vaginalis peritonei.
* The **medial (direct) inguinal hernia** makes its own hernial orifice in the posterior wall of the inguinal canal.

The A. und V. epigastrica inferior form the border between the hernial orifices of the lateral and medial inguinal hernias.

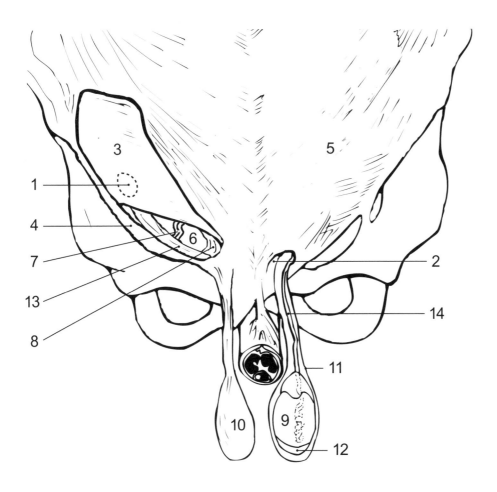

Abb. 5.3

5.4 Inguinal hernias

During its embryonic development, the **testes (1)** descend from their original retroperitoneal location at the level of the kidneys, and reaches the **scrotum (2)** at the point of delivery. Thereby it also everts parts of the abdominal wall which envelop the testes as sheaths, the **Fascia spermatica interna (3)** and **externa (4)**. Where it enters the abdominal wall lateral to the **Vasa epigastrica inferiora (consisting of A. and V. epigastrica inferior, 5)**, the **Annulus inguinalis profundus (deep inguinal ring, 6)** is formed. Further medially lies the exit of the **Annulus inguinalis superficialis (superficial inguinal ring, 7)**. In between them, the **inguinal canal (8)** runs from deep down, laterally and cranially through the abdominal wall like a tunnel to superficial, medial and caudal. Besides the testicular sheath, it also contains other structures which run from or to the testes. These include the **spermatic cord** with the **Ductus deferens (9)** and the Arteria testicularis.

The deep and the superficial inguinal ring as well as the inguinal canal itself represent **physiological weak spots** of the abdominal wall. Here there is a danger of the organs protruding from the abdominal cavity and ending up in the inguinal canal or even in the scrotum. In this case it is called an **inguinal hernia**. There are two forms of inguinal hernias:

Lateral, indirect inguinal hernias (on the left of the illustration below)

In this case, abdominal organs such as **intestinal loops (10)** or parts of the Omentum majus herniate into the inguinal canal or into the scrotum, by taking the same route taken by the testis in its descent. A lateral inguinal hernia benefits from the continued existence of an open **Processus vaginalis peritonei (11a, b)**. This deals with a finger-shaped eversion of the **peritoneum (12a, b**; Peritoneum parietale), which forms next to the testis during the testicular descent and which usually closes completely in the area of the inguinal canal. The **Annulus inguinalis profundus** forms the **internal hernial orifice** in lateral inguinal hernas, lateral (hence the name) of the **Vasa epigastrica inferiora (5a, b)**. Lateral inguinal hernias are mostly **congenital**.

Medial, direct inguinal hernias (on the right of the illustration below)

With this type of inguinal hernia, the **internal hernial orifice** lies medial of the **Vasa epigastrica inferiora (5b)**. The herniating abdominal organs take a direct route through the abdominal wall, thereby everting their wall layers. These then form a **hernial sac (13)** around the herniated organ. Medial inguinal hernias are mostly **acquired** and may only occur later in life with a sharp increase in intra-abdominal pressure.

Clinical remarks

Inguinal hernias can become stuck in the groin or scrotum (incarcerated) on their pathways, e.g. in the area of the internal hernial orifice **(incarceration).** Thereby the blood supply and/or the onward transport of the contents of the intestines can be interrupted. Both can very quickly lead to a necrosis of the herniated organ and to a life-threatening situation, needing urgent surgical intervention.

Women also have an inguinal canal, in that, amongst others, the Ligamentum teres uteri runs from the uterus to the labia majora. The male inguinal canal, however, still presents more of a weak spot due to the number and size of the structures that can pass through the abdominal wall. Correspondingly, inguinal hernias occur nine times more frequently in men than in women.

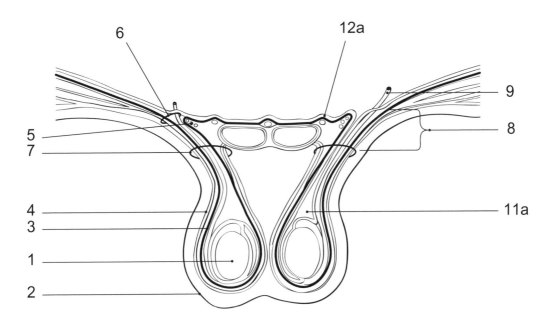

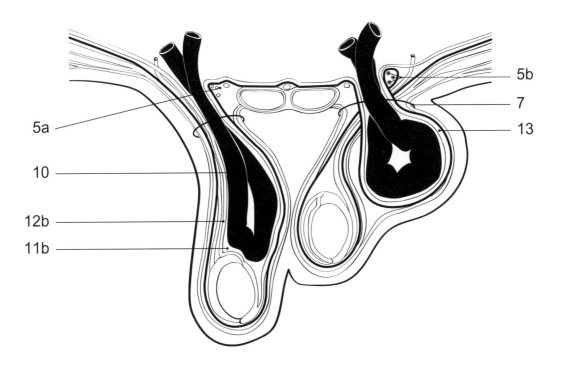

Abb. 5.4

5.5 Upper abdominal organs in situ

After removal of the ventral wall of the torso, the upper abdominal organs become visible (liver, spleen, pancreas, stomach). On the right side of the upper abdomen, below the diaphragm, lies the **liver (hepar, 1),** lifted here to show the **gall bladder (Vesica biliaris, 2)** underneath it.

On the left side of the upper abdomen is the **stomach (gaster, 3)** with its sections:

- **cardia (3a)**
- **fundus (3b)**
- **corpus (3c)**
- **antrum (3d)**
- **pylorus (3e)**

The stomach lies intraperitoneally. The **lesser curvature (Curvatura minor, 3f)** points cranially, the greater curvature **(Curvatura major, 3g)** caudally. From the Curvatura major, the **greater omentum (Omentum majus, 4)** hangs down and hides the small and the large intestine.

Arterial vessel supply of the upper abdominal organs

The upper abdominal organs are supplied from the first unpaired outflow tract of the Aorta abdominalis, the **Truncus coeliacus (5).** The Truncus coeliacus flows out directly underneath the point where the aorta passes through the **diaphragm (6)** in a sagittal direction. It divides immediately thereafter into three branches:

- The **A. gastrica sinistra (7)** runs to the lesser curvature of the stomach. In the area of the cardia, it provides smaller branches to the oesophagus and further along its pathway to the lesser curvature it provides bigger branches to the stomach. It finally anastomoses with the **A. gastrica dextra (8)** from the **A. hepatica communis (9).**
- The **A. hepatica communis (9)** runs in the Lig. hepatoduodenale in the direction of the hepatic porta. It provides the **A. gastrica dextra (8),** which in the Omentum minus (lesser omentum) reaches the lesser curvature of the stomach and there anastomoses with the **A. gastrica sinistra (7).** The **A. gastroduodenalis (10)** is a further branch of the A. hepatica communis. It descends behind the **Pars superior duodeni (11)** and supplies parts of the duodenum and the head of the pancreas. The A. gastroduodenalis also provides the **A. gastroomentalis dextra (12),** running along the greater curvature. Here, branches to the stomach and to the greater omentum branch off. As the last branch of the A. hepatica communis, the **A. hepatica propria (13)** eventually runs in-

to the hepatic porta and provides the liver as the Vas privatum. Before the A. hepatica propria divides itself into respectives branches for the right and the left hepatic lobes, it provides the **A. cystica (14)** to the gall bladder.

- The **A. splenica [lienalis] (15)** gyrates to the left along the upper edge of the pancreas to the spleen, which it supplies. Additionally, it provides numerous branches along its pathway to the corpus and cauda of the pancreas. In the area of the hilum of the spleen, the **A. gastroomentalis sinistra (16)** branches off, anastomosing at the greater curvature with the A. gastroomentalis dextra.

Venous drainage of the upper abdominal organs   The venous blood from the upper abdominal organs flows into the **V. portae (portal vein, 17).** It additionally collects the venous blood of the intestines, runs in the Lig. hepatoduodenale and thereby reaches the hepatic porta. The V. portae capillarises in the liver so that in the area of unpaired abdominal organs two capillary networks are connected consecutively.

The **Ductus choledochus (18)** is the third structure in the Lig. hepatoduodenale. It drains the secretions from the liver and the gall bladder to the duodenum. It reaches the head of the pancreas, dorsally of the Pars superior duodeni, via the Lig. hepatoduodenale and eventually empties into the Pars descendens duodeni (➤ Chap. 5.9).

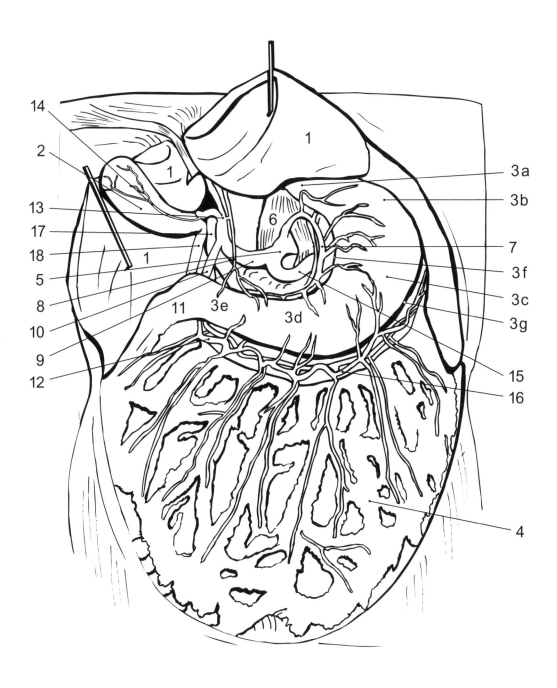

14
2
13
17
18
5
8
10
9
12

1
1
1

6
3e
11
3d

3a
3b
7
3f
3c
3g

15
16

4

Abb. 5.5

99

5.6 Liver

Location and peritoneal relationships   The liver (hepar) lies intraperitoneally in the right upper abdomen below the **diaphragm (1)**. Over the **Area nuda (2)** it is fused with the diaphragm. On the border of the Area nuda, the **Lig. coronarium dextrum (3)** on the right and the **Lig. coronarium sinistrum (4)** on the left connects the liver with the diaphragm. The Lig. coronarium sinistrum runs into the **Appendix fibrosa (5)**. Because of this organisation, the liver moves up and down due to respiration, and is palpable under the right costal arch with deeper inspiration.

Structure   The surface of the liver differentiates the following:
* **Facies diaphragmatica**
* **Facies visceralis**

On the **Facies diaphragmatica** of the liver, the segmentation of the greater **Lobus dexter (6)** and the lesser **Lobus sinister (7)** are visible. Right and left liver lobes are divided by the **Lig. falciforme (8)**. The Lig. falciforme connects the liver with the abdominal wall. The **Lig. teres hepatis (9)** is at the free caudal edge of the Lig. falciforme. This ligament represents the rest of the V. umbilicalis, which runs in the embryonic circulation system from the navel to the hepatic porta.

The gall bladder **(Vesica biliaris, 10a–c)** is ventrally mostly hidden by the liver. Only the **Fundus vesicae biliaris (10a)** sticks out over the caudal edge of the liver.

The **Lobus caudatus (11)** and the **Lobus quadratus (12)** are visible on the **Facies visceralis,** next to the Lobus dexter and the Lobus sinister. They are separated by the structures of the hepatic porta which are arranged in an H-shape. In the hepatic porta, the **V. portae (portal vein, 13)** passes into the liver. As the Vas publicum of the liver it channels the venous blood out of the alimentary canal from the distal oesophagus up to the rectum into the liver, where a second capillarisation takes place. As the Vas privatum of the liver, the **A. hepatica propria (14)** passes into the hepatic porta. There it divides into **A. hepatica dextra (15)** and **A. hepatica sinistra (16)** . The A. hepatica dextra here provides the **A. cystica (17)** to the gall bladder.

Gall bladder   The gall bladder (Vesica biliaris) with its sections is visible to the right of the hepatic porta:
* **Fundus (10a)**
* **Corpus (10b)**
* **Collum (10c)**

The Collum vesicae biliaris continues into the **Ductus cysticus (18)**. The Ductus cysticus merges with the **Ductus hepatici (19)** on the **Ductus choledochus (20)**. The Ductus hepatici and the Ductus choledochus conduct the secretion of the liver, bile, in the direction of the duodenum (➤ Chap. 5.9). The bile can flow via the Ductus cysticus into the gall bladder, where it is stored for use when required. The **V. cava inferior (21)** runs cranially of the gall bladder. It is attached to the liver via the **Lig. venae cavae (22)**.

Fetal circulation   Left of the hepatic porta are the **Lig. teres hepatis (9)** and the **Lig. venosum (23)**. The latter continues the pathway of the V. umbilicalis in the embryonic circulation system as the Ductus venosus and thereby creates a shortcut bypassing the liver to the V. cava inferior and eventually to the right atrium. Postnatally the Ductus venosus closes and is retained as the Lig. venosum.

> **Note**
>
> The liver is both an organ, in which the nutrients which have been absorbed are metabolised, and an exocrine gland. Protein and carbodydrates absorbed from the alimentary canal are conducted to the liver via the V. portae, which capillarises in the liver for a second time. Dietary fats reach the liver indirectly via the Ductus thoracicus (➤ Chap. 4.9) and the body's circulation system.
> The secretion of the liver, bile, is drained into the duodenum via the Ductus hepatici and the Ductus choledochus.

> **Clinical remarks**
>
> Thromboses in the drainage area of the V. portae or pathological changes in the liver (e.g. cirrhosis of the liver) can obstruct the flow of blood in and through the liver, thereby causing **portal hypertension**. The blood then finds other ways to bypass the liver, e.g. as veins in the caudal part of the oesophagus or of the rectum (**portacaval anastomosis,** ➤ Chap. 6.8).

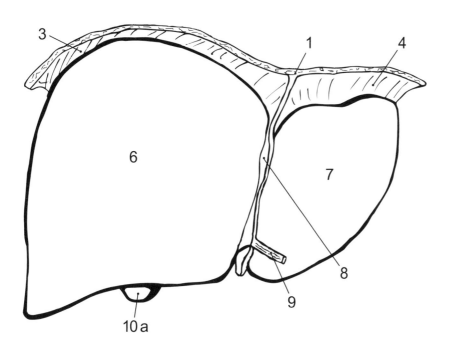

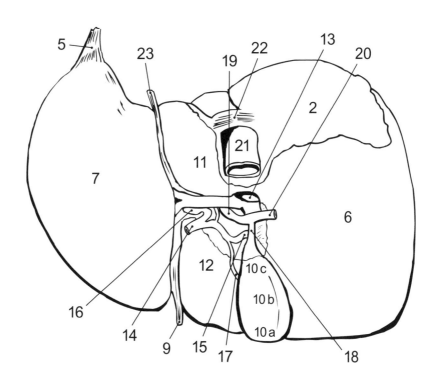

Abb. 5.6

5.7 Portacaval anastomosis

The venous blood of the gastro-intestinal tract flows via the **V. portae hepatis (portal vein, 1)** into the **liver (2).** Thereby the drainage area of the V. portae hepatis encompasses the area of the **cardia of the stomach (3)** up to the **rectum (4)** and also includes the pancreas and the spleen. The V. portae hepatis is formed by the merging of the **Venae mesentericae superior (5)** and **inferior (6)** as well as the **V. lienalis (7).**

If vascular resistance in the liver increases, blood pressure in the portal vein area is raised and leads to **portal hypertension.** Most frequently, the cause of portal hypertension is cirrhosis of the liver, e.g. due to chronic alcohol abuse.

As a result, the portal vein blood flows partially past the liver in the **Vv. cavae superior** or **inferior (8),** where there is the least resistance. Such connections between the drainage areas of the portal vein and the caval vein are called **portacaval anastomosis.**

- In the area of the **cardia of the stomach (3),** blood can flow from the **Vv. gastrici breves (9)** into the **Vv. oesophageae (10).** Via the **Vv. azygos (11)** and **hemiazygos (12)** it eventually reaches the V. cava superior. Because of the increase in blood flow, the Vv. oesophagei expand greatly and **oesophageal varices** are formed. The greatly enlarged veins below the oesophageal mucus membrane in particular present a danger. They can break down and cause life-threatening bleeding in the oesophagus.

- A second portacaval anastomosis can form in the area of the **rectum (4).** Thereby blood flows from the portal venous drainage area from the **Vv. rectales superiores (13)** via the **Plexus venosus rectalis (14)** into the **V. rectalis inferior (15).** The blood flows along the **V. iliaca interna (16)** and eventually into the **V. cava inferior (8).**

- A third portacaval anastomosis can form in the **Ligamentum teres hepatis (17),** which connect the liver with the **navel.** Thereby the blood can flow via the reopened **V. umbilicalis** into the **paraumbilical veins (18)** of the abdominal wall, from where it reaches the upper or lower caval vein via the **Vv. epigastricae superior** or **inferior (19).** When this collateral circulation is strongly marked, the veins of the abdominal wall expand strongly and manifest clinically as Caput medusae.

11 —————
12 —————

10 —————
9 —————
3 —————

2 —————

1 —————

17 —————
5 —————

7 —————

6 —————

18 —————

8 —————

13 —————

16 —————
19 —————

4 —————
14 —————

15 —————

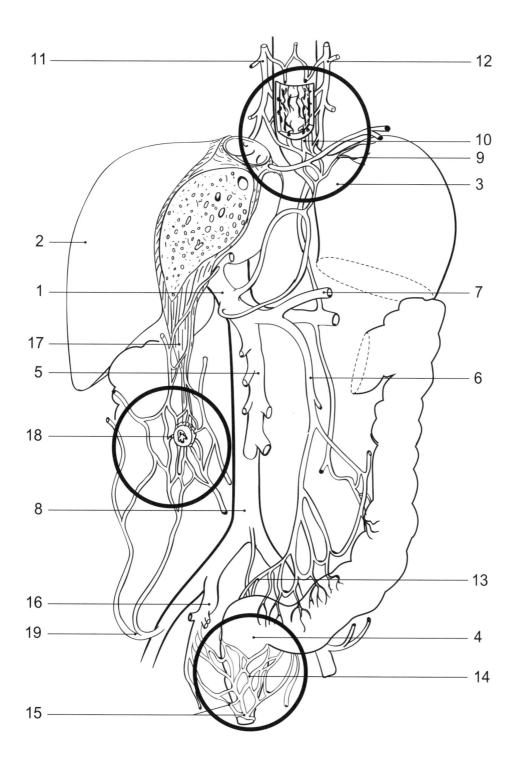

Abb. 5.7

5.8 Retroperitoneal structures of the upper abdomen

The following organs and vessels are located in the retroperitoneum of the upper abdomen:

- **pancreas (1)**
- **duodenum (2),** which encompasses the pancreas in a C-shape
- **kidneys (3a and b)**
- **adrenal glands (Glandulae suprarenales, 4a and b)**
- **abdominal aorta (Aorta abdominalis, 5)** with its branches
- **lower caval vein (V. cava inferior, 6)** with its tributaries
- **portal vein (V. portae hepatis, 7)** with its tributaries

Aorta abdominalis The **Aorta abdominalis (5)** reaches the abdomen via the Hiatus aorticus of the **diaphragm (8)**. There it provides the **Truncus coeliacus (9)** as the first unpaired branch. The Truncus coeliacus divides into:

- the **A. gastrica sinistra (10),** which runs to the lesser curvature of the stomach
- the **A. splenica [lienalis] (11)**, which runs to the left along the upper edge of the pancreas to the spleen
- the **A. hepatica communis (12)**, which lies in the Lig. hepatoduodenale

A. hepatica communis The **A. hepatica communis (12)** runs to the liver after providing the **A. gastroduodenalis (13)** as the **A. hepatica propria (14)**.

The outflow of the **A. mesenterica superior (15)** – the second unpaired branch of the **Aorta abdominalis (5)** – lies hidden behind the body of the pancreas. Further along its path caudally, it is encompassed by the **Proc. uncinatus (1a)** of the pancreas along with the **V. mesenterica superior (16)**. Before the A. mesenterica superior splits into its terminal branches, it provides the **A. pancreaticoduodenalis inferior (17)**. This anastomoses before and behind the head of the pancreas with the **A. pancreaticoduodenalis superior (18)** from the **A. gastroduodenalis (13)**.

V. portae hepatis The confluence of the V. splenica [lienalis] and the V. mesenterica superior with the **portal vein (V. portae hepatis, 7)** lies behind the pancreas. The portal vein drains the venous blood of the gastro-intestinal tract to the liver, which it reaches via the Lig. hepatoduodenale.

In the Lig. hepatoduodenale, next to the **A. hepatica propria (14)** and the V. portae, lies the **Ductus choledochus (19)**, which runs behind the head of the pancreas. It empties into the **Pars descendens (2a) of the duodenum**.

Kidneys and adrenal glands The **adrenal glands (Glandulae suprarenales, 4a and b)** sit on top of the upper poles of the kidneys. The **right adrenal glands (4a)** also lie closely to the **V. cava inferior (6)**.

The **A. renalis (20)** and the **V. renalis (21)** can be seen in the area of the left hilum of the kidneys. The arteries of the kidneys are paired branches of the abdominal aorta. The veins of the kidneys empty into the V. cava inferior. The **ureter (Ureteres, 22a and b)** lie in the area of the hilum of the kidneys furthest dorsally and then descend along the **M. psoas (23)** to the lesser pelvis.

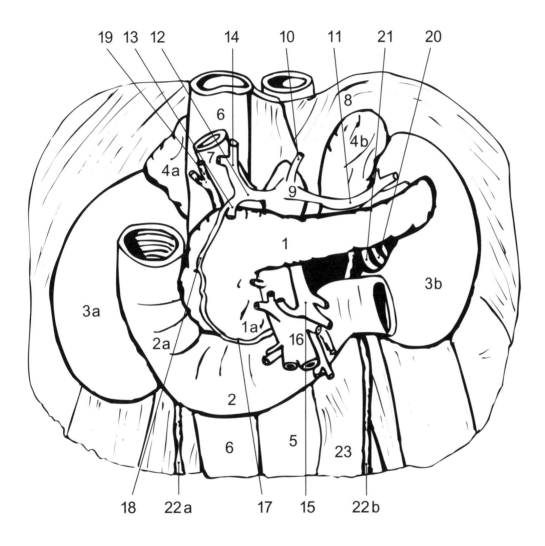

Abb. 5.8

105

5.9 Pancreas

The pancreas lies retroperitoneally in the upper abdomen.
The pancreas consist of:
- a **head (Caput pancreatis, 1a)**
- a **body (Corpus pancreatis, 1b)**
- a **tail (Cauda pancreatis, 1c)**

The **Caput pancreatis (head of the pancreas, 1a)** is surrounded by the **duodenum (2a–c)** in a C-shape. It also has another process, the **Proc. uncinatus (1d)**.

Topography and blood vessel supply   The supply of blood of the pancreas is through the **Truncus coeliacus** and the **A. mesenterica superior (3)**. The A. mesenterica superior descends together with the **V. mesenterica superior (4)** behind the **Pars superior duodeni (2a)** and the head of the pancreas. Here both vessels are also encompassed by the **Proc. uncinatus (1d)**, before running ventrally of the **Pars horizontalis duodeni (2c)**. At the cranial edge of the pancreas runs the **V. splenica [lienalis] (5)** from the spleen to the head of the pancreas. There it merges with the **V. mesenterica superior (4)** at the **V. portae (portal vein, 6)**, ascending to the hepatic porta.

Excretory duct system   The **Ductus choledochus (7)** comes from the hepatic porta. On its way to emtpy into the duodenum, it runs through the head of the pancreas. The **Ductus choledochus (7)** mostly empties together with the **Ductus pancreaticus (duct of Wirsung, 8)** on the **Papilla duodeni major (9)**, which lies in the **Pars descendens duodeni (2b)**. Slightly cranially thereof, the **Ductus pancreaticus accessorius (duct of Santorini, 10)** empties on the **Papilla duodeni minor (11).** The Ductus pancreaticus and pancreaticus accessorius arise from finer branching in the pancreas tail, body and head. They carry the secretion of the pancreas into the duodenum. The Papilla duodeni major uses a sphincter to close.

Clinical remarks

The Ductus choledochus can be compressed by a **carcinoma of the pancreas**. This causes a back-up of bile and thereby a mostly painfree swelling of the gall bladder and jaundice.
Outgoing **gallstones** can get stuck in the Papilla duodeni major, which is a narrow spot in the Ductus choledochus. When the Ductus choledochus and the Ductus pancreaticus empites in the same place, a painful (colic) jaundice occurs, and leads to the pancreas secretion backing up. This can lead to **acute pancreatitis**.

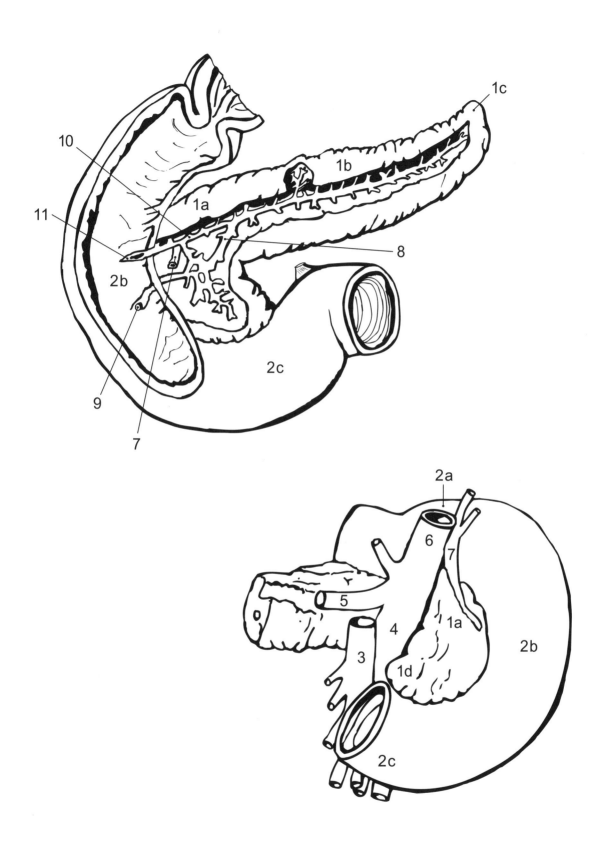

Abb. 5.9

5.10 Kidneys and adrenal glands

The kidneys lie in the retroperitoneal space. The left kidney extends from the 11th rib up to the top of the 3rd lumbar vertebra, the right kidney from the 12th rib to the bottom of the 3rd lumbar vertebra.

The **adrenal glands (Glandulae suprarenales, 1)** lie caplike on top of the kidneys.

Renal fascia and shape of the kidneys   The **renal fascia** of the kidneys are from the superficial to the deep:

- **Fascia renalis**
- **Capsula adiposa**
- **Capsula fibrosa**

The kidney is approx. 12 cm long, 6 cm wide and 3 cm thick. On the **surface** of the kidneys the following are visible:

- **upper pole of the kidney (2)** and **lower pole of the kidney (3)**
- **Margo lateralis (4)**
- **Margo medialis (5)**

Vessel supply   In the area of the Margo medialis, in the **Hilus renalis (6)**, the vessels of the kidney and the ureter run into the kidneys and/or out of these. In the Hilus renalis lies the **A. renalis (7)**, originating from the Aorta abdominalis. Also here is the **V. renalis (8)**, which empties into the V. cava inferior. The **ureter (9)** exits the kidneys dorsally of the vessels.

Longitudinal section through the kidneys   The longitudinal section shows that the Hilus renalis in the kidneys leads into a bigger basin, the **Sinus renalis (10)**. The following branch out in the Sinus renalis:

- the **kidney vessels**
- the **cup-shaped structure of the renal pelvis (Pelvis renalis, 11)**

The kidney parenchyma lies on top of the cup-shaped structure, which subdivides into:

- **renal cortex (Cortex renalis, 12)**
- **renal medulla (Medulla renalis, 13)**

The Medulla renalis consists of the medullary pyramids, with its ridges pointing towards the hilum and with the **Papillae renales (14)** projecting into the **renal calyces (Calices renales, 15)**. Between the medullary pyramids, the column-shaped processes of the renal cortex, the **Columnae renales (16)**, stick out.

Adrenal glands   The **adrenal glands (Glandulae suprarenales, 1)** lie on both sides of the **upper poles of the kidneys (2)** and are separated by the **Capsula adiposa (17)** of the kidneys. The adrenal glands consist of the adrenal medulla, a paraganglion, and the adrenal cortex, an endocrine gland which produces steroid hormones.

The vessel supply of the adrenal glands comes from the **A. suprarenalis superior (18)** from the A. phrenica inferior, the **A. suprarenalis media (19)** from the Aorta abdominalis and the **A. suprarenalis inferior (20)** from the A. renalis.

Clinical remarks

The kidney parenchyma and the efferent urinary passages can be visualised with X-ray imaging and a contrast agent which can be safely used with kidney problems. Shifting of the efferent urinary passage, e.g. by a ureteric stone, presents amongst others as an **enlarged, balloon-like renal pelvicalyceal system**. To make a differential diagnosis, it should be noted that anatomic variants of the calyces present as slim and dendritic, and plump and ampullary.

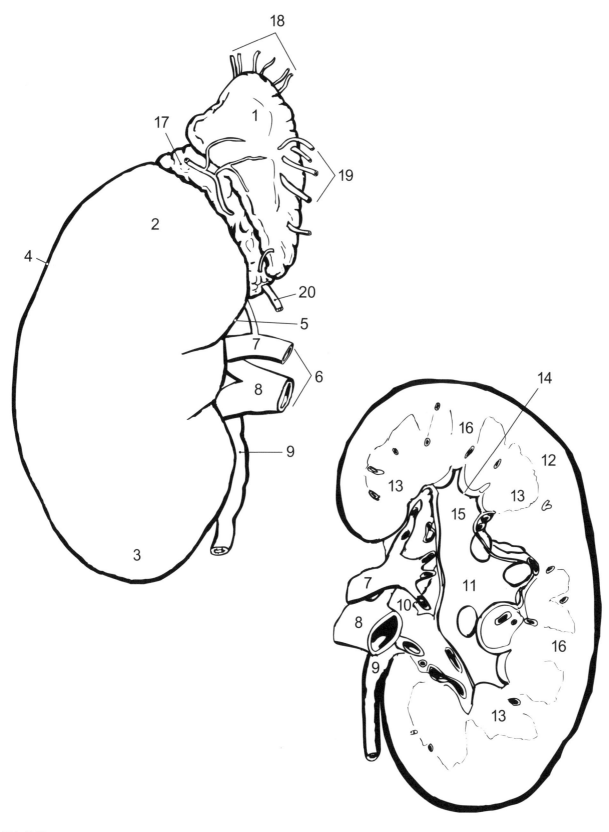

Abb. 5.10

5.11 Intestines and vessel supply

The intestines are divided into:

- **Small intestine (Intestinum tenue)**. This is divided into the:
  - **duodenum**
  - **jejunum (1)**
  - **ileum (2)**
- **Large intestine (Intestinum crassum)**. This is divided into the:
  - **caecum (3)**
  - **appendage of the caecum (Appendix vermiformis, 4)**
  - **colon (Colon ascendens, 5; Colon transversum, 6; Colon descendens, Colon sigmoideum)**
  - **rectum**

The **jejunum (1)** begins at the **Flexura duodenojejunalis (7)**. It passes into the **ileum (2)**. Macroscopically, the jejunum and the ileum are indistinguishable and continue as one without interruption. While the duodenum is not visible retroperitoneally, the position of the jejunum and the ileum is intraperitoneal. Their **mesentery (8)** originates from the back abdominal wall with a broad root. It begins on the right side approx. at the level of the iliosacral joint, ascends to the left and ends up at the 2nd lumbar vertebra. The terminal ileum empties end-to-side in the colon.

Caudal of this inflow, a blind end of the colon is thereby formed, the **caecum (3)**. The **Appendix vermiformis (4)** emerges from here. Cranial of the inflow of the ileum, the colon continues with the **Colon ascendens (5)** and the **Colon transversum (6)**. The Appendix vermiformis and the Colon transversum lie intraperitoneally and contain the **Mesocolon transversum (9)**.

The position of the caecum can vary from lying either retroperitoneally (Caecum fixum) or intraperitoneally. A very distinctive variant is called a Mobile Caecum.

The Colon ascendens lies retroperitoneally. Macroscopically, the colon can be differentiated from the small intestine through the transverse grooves and the **haustra (10)** which lie between them and the longitudinal thickenings of the colon musculature, the **teniae**. In this view, the **Taenia libera (11)** are visible.

Vessel supply The vessel supply of the Flexura duodenojejunalis up to and including the Colon transversum comes from the **A. mesenterica superior (12)**. It is the second unpaired outflow of the Aorta abdominalis and initially runs retroperitoneally behind the pancreas (➤ Chap. 5.9). Caudal of the pancreas, it enters the root of the mesentery and branches out into approx. 15–20 **Aa. jejunales and ileales (13),** which supply the small intestine. The Aa. jejunales and ileales inside the mesentery branch out further and are connected to each other through anastomising arterial arches.

The **A. ileocolica (14)** is at the attachment point of the root of the mesentery and runs parallel to it. It supplies the terminal Ileum and also provides branches to the caecum, as well as the **A. appendicularis** to the Appendix vermiformis.

The next outflow of the A. mesenterica superior is the **A. colica dextra (15)** which supplies the Colon ascendens. It anastomoses in the area of the right flexure of the colon with the **A. colica media (16)**, which runs in the Mesocolon transversum and supplies the Colon transversum.

Note

Intestine section	Blood Vessel supply
duodenum	Aa. pancreaticoduodenales superiores anteriores and posteriores from the A. gastroduodenalis and the A. pancreaticoduodenalis inferior from the A. mesenterica superior
jejunum	Aa. jejunales from the A. mesenterica superior
ileum	Aa. ileales from the A. mesenterica superior
terminal ileum	A. ileocolica from the A. mesenterica superior
caecum	Aa. caecales anterior and posterior from the A. ileocolica
Appendix vermiformis	A. appendicularis from the A. ileocolica
Colon ascendens	A. colica dextra from the A. mesenterica superior
Colon transversum	A. colica media from the A. mesenterica superior
Colon decendens	A. colica sinistra from the A. mesenterica inferior
Colon sigmoideum	Aa. sigmoideae from the A. mesenterica inferior

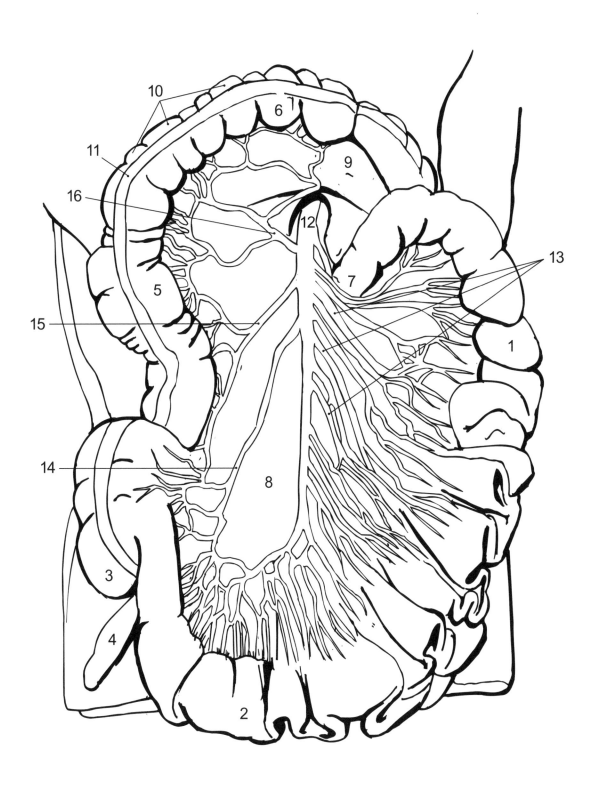

Abb. 5.11

111

5.12 Pathways of the retroperitoneal space

The **M. quadratus lumborum (1)** and the **M. psoas major (2)** form the muscular border of the back abdominal wall.

Nerves   The **N. subcostalis (3)** and the nerves of the Plexus lumbalis lie between the roots of the M. psoas major. In the craniocaudal direction, running laterally via the M. quadratus lumborum and/or the **M. iliacus (4)**:

* **N. subcostalis (3)**
* **N. iliohypogastricus (5)**
* **N. ilioinguinalis (6)**
* **N. cutaneus femoris lateralis (7)**

The Nn. subcostalis, iliohypogastricus and ilioinguinalis penetrate into the M. transversus abdominis and run between it and the M. obliquus abdominis in an arch ascending to ventral.

On the M. psoas major, the **N. genitofemoralis (8)** runs to caudal and branches out into its terminal branches, the **Rr. genitalis (8a)** and **femoralis (8b)**.

The **N. femoralis (9)** lies in the groove between the M. psoas major and the M. iliacus. It runs to caudal and passes underneath the inguinal ligament through the Lacuna musculorum on the thigh. As the only nerve of the Plexus lumbalis, the **N. obturatorius (10)** runs medially of the M. psoas major along the wall of the lesser pelvis to the Canalis obturatorius.

The abdominal part of the **Truncus sympathicus (11)** descends paramedially along the front of the vertebrae.

Arteries   The **Aorta abdominalis (12)** passes through the Hiatus aorticus. It provides the following branches:

* **Aa. phrenicae inferiores**
* **Truncus coeliacus (unpaired, 13)**
* **Aa. suprarenales mediae**
* **A. mesenterica superior (unpaired, 14)**
* **Aa. renales (15)**
* **Aa. ovaricae and/or Aa. testiculares (16)**
* **A. mesenterica inferior (unpaired, 17)**

The Aorta abdominalis divides into both the **Aa. iliacae communes** in front of the 4th lumbar vertebra **(18a and b)**.

Veins   To the right of the Aorta abdominalis lies the **V. cava inferior (19)**. It is formed by the confluence of both the **Vv. iliacae communes (20a and b)** at the approximate level of the 5th lumbar vertebra.

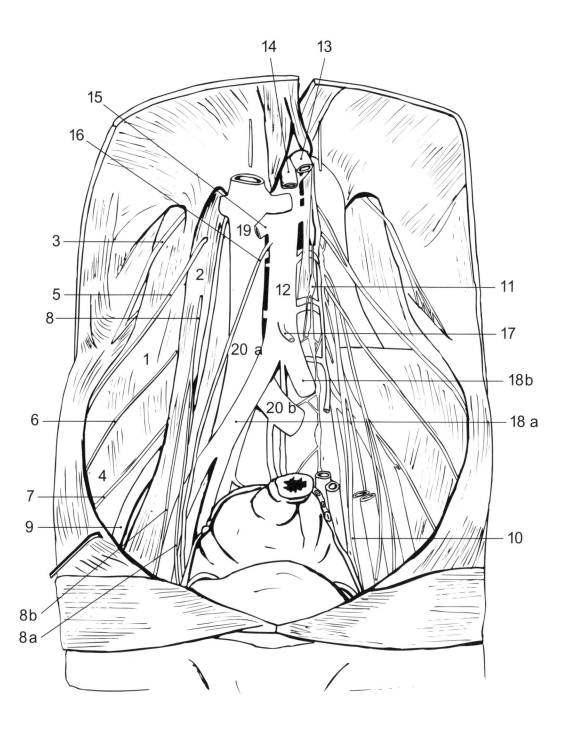

Abb. 5.12

5.13 Plexus lumbalis

The Plexus lumbalis is formed by the Rr. anteriores of the spinal cord segments Th12–L4. To help with orientation, the vertebrae have been marked LI–LV.

The Plexus lumbalis consists of the following branches:

- **N. iliohypogastricus (1, Th12–L1)**
- **N. ilioinguinalis (2, Th12–L1)**
- **N. genitofemoralis (3, L1–3)**
- **N. cutaneus femoris lateralis (4, L2–3)**
- **N. femoralis (5, L2–4)**
- **N. obturatorius (6, L2–4)**

The upper branches, the **N. iliohypogastricus (1, Th12–L1)** and the **N. ilioinguinalis (2, Th12–L1)**, often originate from a common stem and divide further along. They are involved in the innervation of the abdominal muscles. The N. ilioinguinalis also provides sensory innervation on the skin of the inguinal region and the scrotum.

The **N. genitofemoralis (3, L1–2)** divides into:

- the **R. femoralis**, which runs through the Lacuna vasorum to the proximal, ventral thigh, there supplying the skin, and
- the **R. genitalis**, which also runs through the inguinal canal and there innervates the M. cremaster and the scrotum.

The **N. cutaneus femoris lateralis (4, L2–3)** descends, penetrates the inguinal ligament at the level of the Spina iliaca anterior superior and innervates the skin on the lateral thigh.

The **N. femoralis (5, L2–4)** reaches the thigh through the Lacuna musculorum. It innervates the skin of the ventral thigh, the M. quadriceps femoris and the M. sartorius. Its terminal branch, the **N. saphenus**, innervates the skin on the medial lower leg.

The **N. obturatorius (6, L2–4)** runs as the only nerve of the Plexus lumbalis medially along the wall of the lesser pelvis to the Canalis obturatorius. It reaches the medial side of the thigh through it, where it supplies the skin and the muscles of the adductor group.

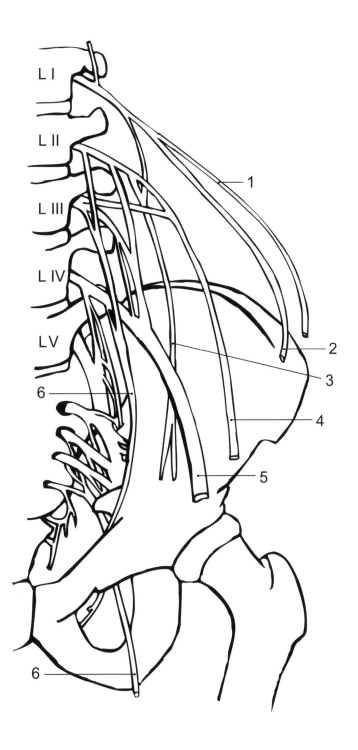

L I

L II

L III

L IV

L V

6

6

1

2

3

4

5

Abb. 5.13

6.1 Pelvic floor

The pelvic floor is bounded ventrally by both the lower **pubic bone branches (Rr. inferiores ossis pubis, 1)** and the **symphysis (2)**, lateral of both the **ischial tuberosities (Tuber ischiadicum, 3)** and the **Ligg. sacrotuberalia (4)** as well as dorsally of the apex of the **Os sacrum (sacral bone, 5)**. The pelvic outlet is closed by the **pelvic floor,** an occlusion mechanism consisting of muscles and fascia. The striated musculature of the pelvic floor and its fascial parts carry the pelvic organs and are important for fecal and urinary continence. There are two muscle plates in the pelvic floor:

- **Diaphragma pelvis (6)**
- **Diaphragma urogenitale (7)**

View from caudal   The **Diaphragma pelvis** is formed by the **M. levator ani (8)** and the **M. coccygeus (9)**. The M. levator ani runs in a U-shape from the dorsal side of the pubic bone and from a tendinous sheet which extends along the pelvic wall. Ventrally it leaves a gap, the **Hiatus urogenitalis**. Both the muscles of the M. levator ani enfold the **rectum** and the **anus (10)**, which here passes through the pelvic floor. The anus is circularly surrounded by the **M. sphincter ani externus (11)**. Dorsal of the anus, the M. levator ani is connected via the **Lig. anococcygeum (12)** with the Os sacrum.

The **Diaphragma urogenitale (7)** which runs transversely between the lower **pubic bone branches (1),** closes the Hiatus genitalis.

The Diaphragma urogenitale consists of the muscle plate of the **M. transversus perinei profundus (13)** and the narrow **M. transversus perinei superficialis (14)**. The Diaphragma urogenitale contains the **openings for the urethra (15)** as well as for the **vagina (16)** in women. Around the opening of the urethra are the circularly-running fibres of the **M. sphincter urethrae externus (17)**.

In front of the anus and dorsally of the Diaphragma urogenitale is a fascial plate, the **Centrum tendineum perinei (18)**.

View from cranial   In this view the different sections of the M. levator ani can be seen. It consists of four muscles:

- **M. puborectalis**
- **M. pubococcygeus (19)**
- **M. pubovaginalis** (only in women)
- **M. levator prostatae** (only in men)
- **M. iliococcygeus (20a and b)**

The **M. pubococcygeus (19)** originates from the dorsal side of the pubic bone and runs in a U-shaped loop around the rectum.

Thereby it remains open ventrally of the **Hiatus urogenitalis (21)**. The M. pubococcygeus forms the so-called levator ani muscle which surrounds the rectum. It is the most important sphinctre of the anus.

The **M. iliococcygeus (20a and b)** originates at a tendinous sheet, the **Arcus tendineus musculi levatoris ani (22)**, which runs on the inside of the lesser pelvis and also spans the M. obturatorius internus. The M. iliococcygeus attaches laterally to the M. pubococcygeus.

The **M. coccygeus (23a und b)** attach dorsally of the M. levator ani. It originates at the Spina ischiadica and runs to the Os coccygis.

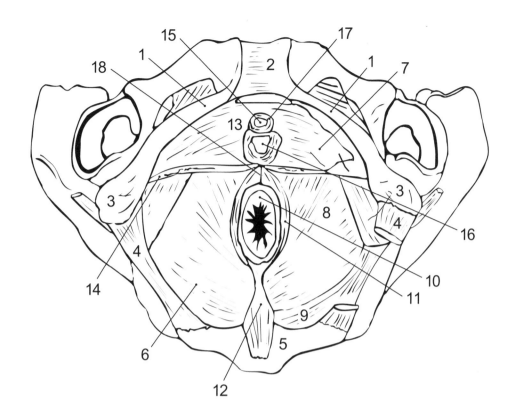

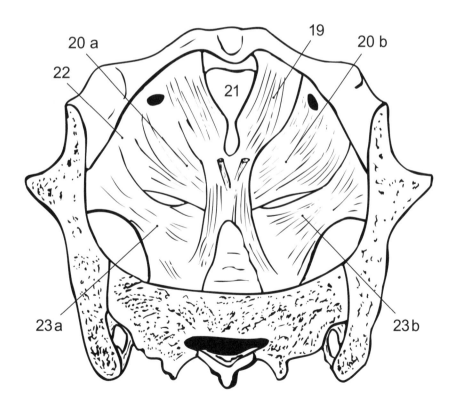

Abb. 6.1

6.2 Pelvic floor in women

Muscles of the pelvic floor The following belong to the lower layer of the pelvic floor:

- **M. transversus perinei superficialis (1)**
- **M. sphincter ani externus (2)**, ➤ Chap. 6.1
- **M. bulbospongiosus (3)**
- **M. ischiocavernosus (4)**

The **M. bulbospongiosus** encompasses the **Vestibulum vaginae (5)** and inserts ventrally of the **clitoris (6)**.

The **Mm. ischiocavernosi** lies near the ends of the pubic bone and covers the **Corpus cavernosum clitoridis (7)** on both sides. With sexual arousal, they carry the blood ventrally in the direction of the cavernous body.

Innervation The striated muscles of the pelvic floor are innervated by the **N. pudendus (8a and b)** from the **Plexus pudendalis (S2–4)** and from direct branches from the **Plexus sacralis**. The N. pudendus leaves the pelvis through the Foramen infrapiriforme, curves directly back around the Spina ischiadica into the Foramen ischiadicum minus and thereby reaches the **Fossa ischioanalis (9)**.

The **Fossa ischioanalis** is a pyramidal space between the wall of the lesser pelvis on the one side and the pelvic floor on the other side. Its base is directed to the surface of the perineum, its apex to the symphysis. The lateral wall of the Fossa ischiorectalis is bounded by the M. obturatorius internus.

The pupendal canal, the anatomical structure in the pelvis through which the N. pudendus runs to the pelvic floor, branches out and innervates the pelvic floor musculature, as well as the surface of the perineum and the outer genitalia.

Blood Vessel supply The vessel supply of the pelvic floor and the perineum is carried out via the **A. and V. pudenda interna (10a and b)**, which have the same pathway as the **N. pudendus (8)**. The A. pudenda interna originates from the A. iliaca interna. The V. pudenda empties into the V. iliaca interna.

Clinical remarks

For surgical intervention in the area of the perineum, **conductive anaesthesia of the N. pudendus** can be carried out. Herein the Spina ischiadica is located via the vagina and the anaesthetic is injected around it.

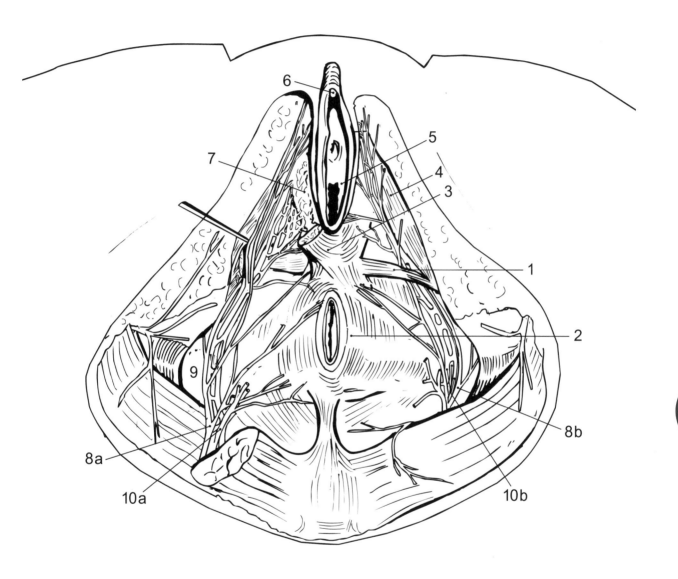

Abb. 6.2

6.3 Pelvic floor in men

Muscles of the pelvic floor   The bottom layer of the pelvic floor is formed by the same muscles in both men and women:

- **M. transversus perinei superficialis (1)**
- **M. sphincter ani externus (2)**, ➤ Chap. 6.1
- **M. bulbospongiosus (3)**
- **M. ischiocavernosus (4)**

The pathway and the function of the Mm. bulbospongiosus and ischiocavernosus differ in men from women.

The **M. bulbospongiosus (3)** originates from the Diaphragma urogenitale, at the Sphincter ani externus and at the median raphe of the pelvic floor. It runs obliquely to the front and surrounds the Bulbus corporis cavernosi in a circular shape. The M. bulbospongiosus shortens and narrows the urethra and empties it intermittently.

The **M. ischiocavernosus (4)** runs closely along the ends of the pubic bone and arises from the crus of the Corpus cavernosum penis. It surrounds the cavernous body and attaches to the front of its Tunica albuginea. On this dorsum of the cavernous body, the fibres of both sides converge in a loop. The M. ischiocavernosus helps with the erection and supports ejaculation.

Innervation and vessel supply   The nerve and vessel supply of the perineum, of the pelvic floor and of the outer genitalia are carried out by the **N. pudendus (5)**, the **A. pudenda interna (6)** and the **V. pudenda interna (7)**, taking the same pathway as described for women.

Clinical remarks

Erectile dysfunction can be caused by damage to the N. pudendus as well as by circulatory disorders in the area of the A. pudenda interna.

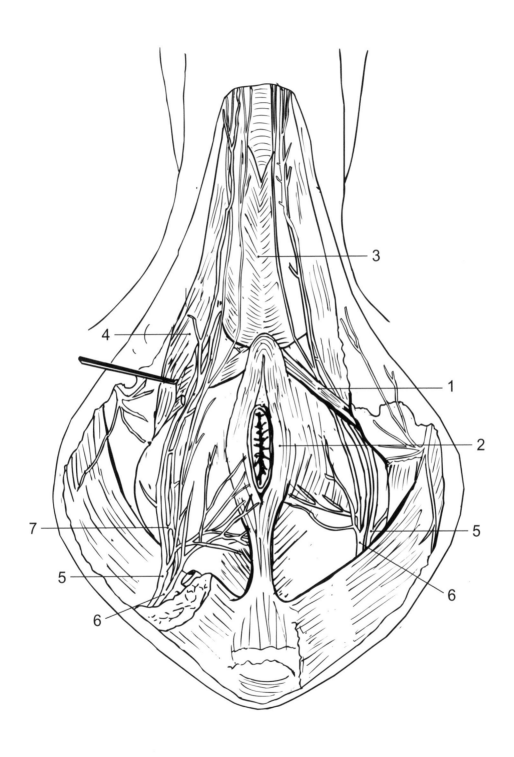

Abb. 6.3

6.4 Sagittal section through the female pelvis

The positional relationships of the pelvic organs are especially clear in the median sagittal section. The ventral border of the lesser pelvis forms the **symphysis (1)**, and the dorsal border forms the **Os coccygis (2)** and the **Os sacrum (3)**.

Urinary bladder   The **urinary bladder (Vesica urinaria, 4)** abuts the symphysis dorsally. The sections of the urinary bladder are:
- **Corpus vesicae (4a)**
- **Apex vesicae (4b)**
- **Fundus vesicae (4c)**
- **Collum vesicae (4d)**

The obliterated **urachus (5)** ascends from the Apex vesicae to the navel. The Apex vesicae is covered cranially by the **Peritoneum parietale (6)** and thereby lies sub- and/or preperitoneally. In front of the urinary bladder is the **Spatium retropubicum (7)**, which is filled with loose connective tissue. The urinary bladder expands gradually when filled, raises the Peritoneum parietale cranially and ends up above the **symphysis (1)** directly dorsal of the abdominal wall. The approx. 4–5 cm long female **urethra (8)** leaves from the Collum vesicae (4d). It penetrates the pelvic floor and empties in the area of the **Vestibulum vaginae (9)**.

Uterus   The **uterus (womb, 10)** lies dorsally over the bladder. The sections of the uterus are visible: cranial is the **Fundus uteri (10a)**, with the **Corpus uteri (10b)** adjoining as well as the **Isthmus uteri (10c)** and the **Cervix uteri (10d)** furthest caudal.

The Cervix uteri projects into the **vagina (11)** with the **Portio vaginalis (10e)**. The vagina encompasses the Portio vaginalis, so that ventrally and dorsally a gap is formed between the vaginal wall and the Portio vaginalis: the **ventral and dorsal vaginal vault (12a and b)**. The position of the uterus over the urinary bladder is brought about by the **anteversion** (ventral inclination of the uterus to the transverse line) and the **anteflexio** (angle between the cervix and the Corpus uteri).

Rectum   The **rectum (13)** adjoins dorsally of the uterus. The rectum nestles into the cranial part of the kyphosis of the **Os sacrum (3)** (Flexura sacralis) and then turns in a ventral direction (Flexura perinealis) at the opening into the pelvic floor. In the rectum the biggest of three transverse folds, **Kohlrausch's fold**, projects from the right into the lumen of the rectum. Below this fold, the rectum extends to the **Ampulla recti (13a)**. The **Canalis analis (13b)** joins caudally of the Ampulla recti and eventually passes through the pelvic floor.

Peritoneal relationships   The Peritoneum parietale of the abdominal wall runs via the **Apex vesicae (4b)** and then turns over on the **Corpus uteri (10b)**. Thereby the **Excavatio vesicouterina (14)** is formed between the urinary bladder and the uterus. The peritoneum then runs further via the **Fundus uteri (10a)**, completely covers the uterus on the dorsal side and reaches the posterior vaginal vault. There the peritoneum turns over on the rectum. Thereby the **Excavatio rectouterina (15, clinical description: Douglas space)** is formed between the uterus and the rectum. It represents the deepest point of the peritoneal cavity in women.

Clinical remarks

A full urinary bladder can be punctured above the symphysis through the abdominal wall, without having to open the peritoneal cavity. Deviations from the position of the uterus can impact negatively on **conception**.

Due to the peritoneal relationships in the area of the Excavatio rectouterina, the peritoneal cavity of the woman can be punctured through the vagina and the posterior vaginal vault.

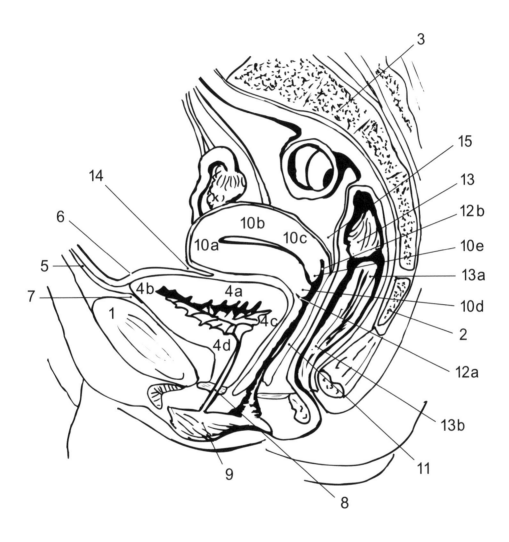

Abb. 6.4

123

6.5 Sagittal section through the male pelvis

In the median sagittal section, through the lesser pelvis, the **symphysis (1)** can be seen forming the ventral border and also the **Os sacrum (2)** and the **Os coccygis (3)**, forming the dorsal border.

The positional relationships of the pelvic organs are clearly represented in this incision.

Urinary bladder The position and the sections of the **urinary bladder (Vesica urinaria, 4)** correspond with those of the woman (➤ Chap. 6.4). The **urethra (5)** of the man starts at the Collum vesicae with the Pars prostatica. It runs here through the **Prostata (6)** which lies below the bladder neck and above the pelvic floor. Subsequently, the Pars perinealis of the urethra passes through the **Diaphragma urogenitale (7)** and then runs as the Pars spongiosa through the **Corpus spongiosum (8)** of the penis. It empties in the area of the Glans penis in the **Fossa navicularis (9)**. The **Corpus cavernosum penis (10),** the cavernous body of the penis, is also visible.

Rectum The position, sections and inner surface of the **rectum (11)** correspond to those of the woman (➤ Chap. 6.4).

Peritoneal relationships The Peritoneum parietale of the abdominal wall runs across the Apex vesicae and turns over on the rectum. In the area where it turns over lies the **Gl. vesiculosa** (seminal vesicle, not shown) dorsal of the **urinary bladder (4)**. The urinary bladder also lies subperitoneally.

Where it transitions to the Colon sigmoideum, the **rectum (11)** displays a short mesentery and can thereby lie intraperitoneally. Further caudal in the area of Kohlrausch's fold and the Flexura perinealis, the rectum is covered ventrally by the Peritoneum parietale, and thereby lies here retroperitoneally. Below the Flexura perinealis the rectum no longer has any connection to the peritoneum. Due to this peritoneal pathway, the **Excavatio rectovesicalis (12),** the deepest point of the male peritoneal cavity, is formed here between the rectum and the urinary bladder.

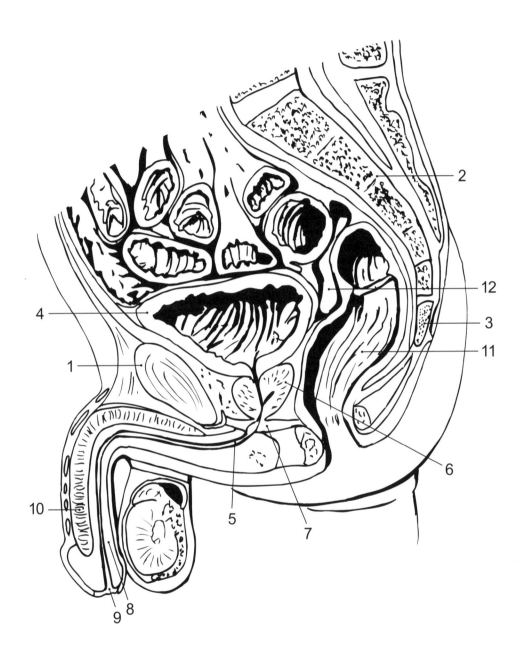

Abb. 6.5

125

6.6 Pathways of the pelvis

After preparing the pelvic viscera in the median sagittal section, the pelvic floor and the pathways of the pelvis are visible. Of the pelvic floor, the **M. levator ani** with its parts, the **M. pubococcygeus (1)** and the **M. iliococcygeus (2),** as well as the **M. coccygeus (3)**, can be seen.

Innervation   On the ventral side of the Os sacrum, the **Plexus sacralis (5)** is formed through the merging of the **Rr. anteriores of the sacral myelomeres (4).** It here provides direct branches to innervate the Diaphragma pelvis.

Of the **Plexus lumbalis,** the **R. genitalis of the N. genitofemoralis (6)**, which passes through the **Anulus inguinalis profundus (7)** into the inguinal canal, can be seen. The **R. femoralis of the N. genitofemoralis (8)** runs with the **A. iliaca externa (9)** through the Lacuna vasorum to the upper thigh.

A. iliaca interna   The vessel supply of the pelvic wall and viscera is provided by branches of the A. iliaca interna. This comes about because the **A. iliaca communis (10)** splits into the **A. iliaca externa (9)** and the **A. iliaca interna (11)**. Five parietal and five visceral branches of the A. iliaca interna can be seen.

The five **parietal branches** supply the pelvic wall:

- **A. iliolumbalis (12)** runs posterior of the M. psoas major ascending to lateral.
- **A. obturatoria (13)** runs along the Linea terminalis ventrally and passes through the Canalis obturatorius together with the N. obturatorius to the medial side of the upper thigh.
- **A. sacralis lateralis (14)** descends anterior of the Foramina sacralia anteriora of the Os sacrum.
- **A. glutea superior (15)** passes through the Foramen suprapiriforme from the pelvis and thereby reaches the gluteal area.
- **A. glutea inferior (16)** leaves the pelvis through the Foramen infrapiriforme and thereby reaches the gluteal area.

The **five visceral** branches supply the pelvic viscera:

- **A. umbilicalis** ascends in the fetus on the abdominal wall to the navel and from there via the umbilical cord further along to the placenta. Postnatally the cranial part obliterates and only the initial part remains intact as the **A. vesicalis superior (17)**.
- **A. vesicalis inferior (18)** runs to the Fundus vesicae, to the prostate and to the Glandulae vesiculosa.
- **A. pudenda interna (19)** leaves the pelvis via the Foramen infrapiriforme, curves around the Spina ischiadica and passes back through the Foramen ischiadicum minus into

the pelvis. In the Fossa ischioanalis it branches out and supplies the pelvic floor, the perineum and the outer genitalia.

- **A. rectalis media**   (not shown) supplies the rectum (➤ Chap. 6.7).
- **A. uterina** (not shown) supplies the uterus (➤ Chap. 6.9).

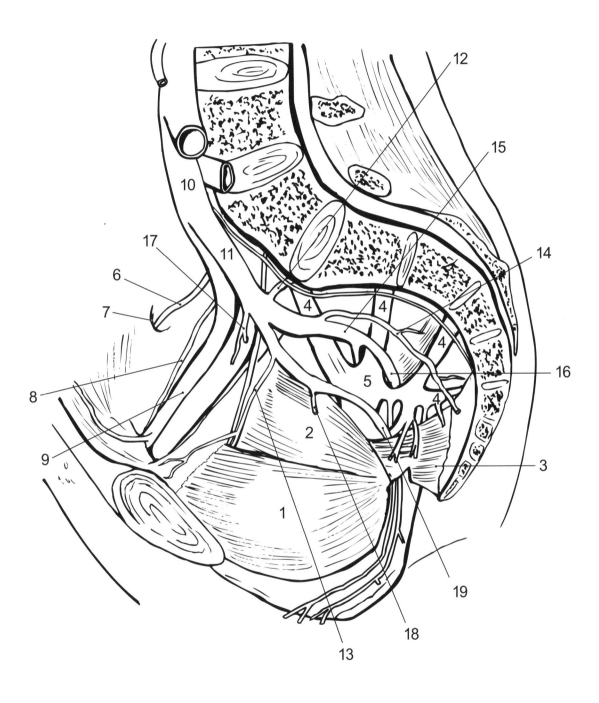

Abb. 6.6

6.7 Arteries of the rectum

There are primarily three arteries that supply the rectum:

- The **A. rectalis superior (1)** originates from the 3rd and most caudal unpaired outflow tract of the **Aorta abdominalis (2),** the **A. mesenterica inferior (3)**. After providing the **Aa. sigmoideae (4),** the A. rectalis superior reaches the rectum as a terminal branch of the A. mesenterica inferior. The supply area of the A. mesenterica inferior extends from the left colon flexure up to the rectum. The **A. rectalis superior** supplies the cranial sections of the rectum including those of the Ampulla recti. Its terminal branches penetrate the muscle layers of the retum and feed the Corpus cavernosum recti. The **Corpus cavernosum recti** is a cavernous body in the area of the anal canal, which serves as a gas- and water-tight closure of the anus.
- The **A. rectalis media (5)** is a visceral branch of the **A. iliaca interna (6)**. It is situated in the area of the caudal Ampulla recti at the rectum und supplies it.
- The **A. rectalis inferior (7)** is a branch of the **A. pudenda interna (8)**, which thereby represents a visceral outflow of the **A. iliaca interna (6)**. It supplies the outer sections of the anal canal and the sphinctres of the anus.

Clinical remarks

The arteries of the rectum all form anastomoses with each other, so that with a surgical ligation of the A. rectalis superior the supply of the rectum is still ensured. Pathological extensions of the Corpus cavernosum recti are known as haemorrhoids. Blood from **haemorrhoids** is bright red, as the Corpus cavernosum recti is supplied with arterial blood from the A. rectalis superior.

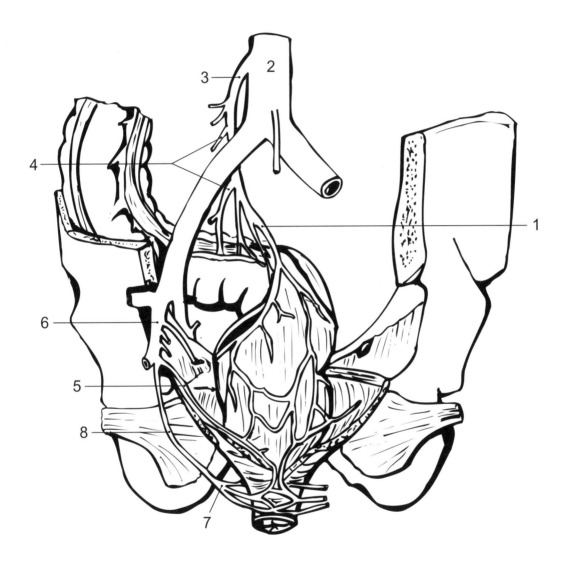

Abb. 6.7

129

6.8 Veins of the rectum

The veins of the rectum drain in two different directions:
- via the **V. mesenterica inferior (1) to the V. portae**
- to the **V. cava inferior (2)**

Around the rectum there is a large venous plexus, the **Plexus venosus rectalis (3)**. From the venous plexus, the blood can drain cranially via the **V. mesenterica inferior (1)** into the portal vein (V. portae) and thereby into the liver.

Alternatively, there are drainage paths to the **V. iliaca interna (7)** via the **V. rectalis media (4)** as well as to the **V. rectalis inferior (5)** and the **V. pudenda interna (6).** Eventually the blood flows into the **V. cava inferior (2)** via the **V. iliaca communis (8)**.

The venous plexus of the rectum therefore presents a border between the drainage areas of the V. portae and the V. cava inferior **(portacaval anastomosis)** .

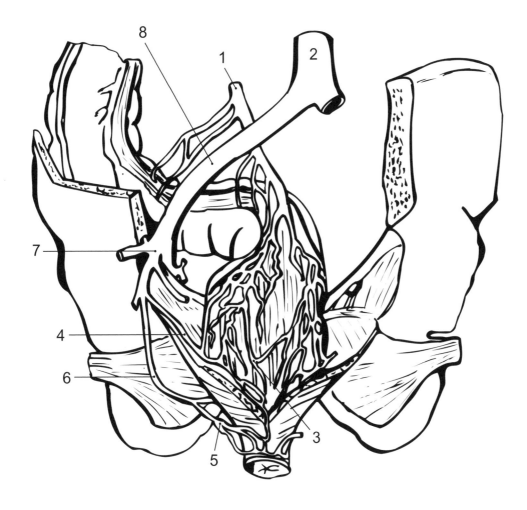

Abb. 6.8

6.9 Uterus and appendages and their blood vessel supply

Uterus (womb, 1), Tuba uterina (Fallopian tube, 2) und **Ovarium (ovary, 3)** lie intraperitoneally. They are covered by the peritoneum and are connected to the pelvic wall via their ligaments. The depiction shows the following sections of the uterus:

- **Fundus uteri (1a)**
- **Corpus uteri (1b)**
- **Cervix uteri (1c)**

The Cervix uteri is surrounded by the muscular sleeve of the **vagina (4)**. The Tuba uterina flows into the uterus in the area of the tubular angle between the Fundus uteri and the Corpus uteri. From here the **Lig. teres uteri (5)** also runs to the inguinal canal.

Blood Vessels In the area of the Cervix uteri, the **A. uterina (6)** passes the uterus closely. It comes as a visceral branch of the A. iliaca interna from the pelvic wall and runs in the base of the **Lig. latum (7)**, the ligament of the uterus, to the cervix. Here it provides the **Rr. vaginales (8)** to the vagina. Subsequently it winds upwards laterally of the uterus and provides the **R. tubarius (9)** at the tubular drainage angle. This branch runs in the ligament of the Tuba uterina, the **Mesosalpinx (10)**, in the direction of the ovary.

The **A. ovarica (11)** runs from cranial to the ovary as a branch of the Aorta abdominalis via the **Lig. suspensorium ovarii (12)**. In the area of the **mesovarium (13)** and the **mesosalpinx (10)** it anastomoses with the **R. ovaricus (14)** of the **A. uterina**.

Clinical remarks

With surgical removal of the uterus, i.e. **hysterectomy,** and during ligation of the A. uterina, it is important on the one hand to take into account the close proximity to the urethra in the area of the Cervix uteri, and on the other hand its anastomosis with the A. ovarica in the area of the tube which also needs to be ligated.

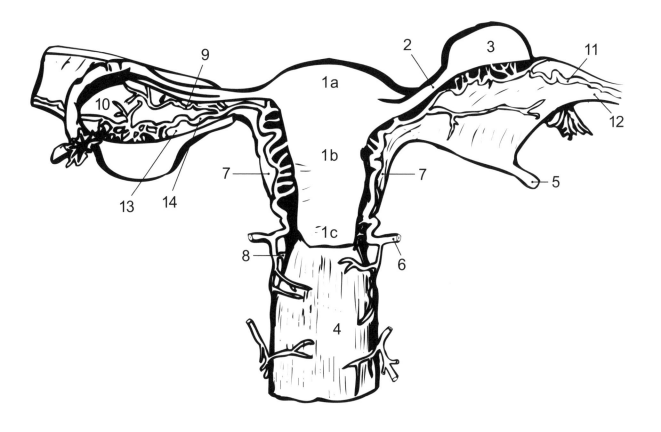

Abb. 6.9

133

6.10 Uterus and appendages

Uterus   After opening up the **uterus (1),** the following sections become visible:

- **Fundus uteri (1a)**
- **Corpus uteri (1b)**
- **Isthmus uteri (1c)**
- **Cervix uteri (1d)**

The Cervix uteri projects with its **Portio vaginalis (1e)** into the **vagina (2).** Thereby a gap is formed between the vaginal wall and the Portio vaginalis, the **vaginal vault (3).** Below the **peritoneal coating of the uterus (4)** lies the thick muscular layer of the uterine wall, the **myometrium (5).**

Tuba uterina   In the area of the **tubular drainage angle (6),** the **Tuba uterina (Fallopian tube, 8)** flows into the uterus. It shows four sections:

- **Infundibulum tubae uterinae (tube funnel, 8a)**
- **Ampulla tubae uterinae (8b)**
- **Isthmus tubae uterinae (8c)**
- **Pars uterina tubae**

The Tuba uterina begins at the **ovary (7)** with the Infundibulum tubae uterinae, which is encompassed by the **Fimbriae tubae uterinae (8d).** The Infundibulum tubae uterinae passes into the **Ampulla tubae uterinae (8b).** It joins the narrow **Isthmus tubae uterinae (8c),** which ends at the intramural section of the tube in the area of the tubal drainage angle.

The **epoophoron (9)** in the mesosalpinx and the **paroophoron (10)** which lies between the epoophoron and the uterus, are visible as remnants of the mesonephros.

Endopelvic fascia of the uterus   The endopelvic fascia, the retaining ligaments of the uterus, consist primarily of:

- **Lig. teres uteri (11)**
- **Lig. latum uteri (12)**
- **Lig. cardinale (13)**
- **Lig. sacrouterinum (14)**

On the left side of the illustration, only parts of the endopelvic fascia of the uterus are visible. The **Lig. teres uteri (11)** runs from the tubal angle to the inguinal canal. The **Lig. ovarii proprium (15)** runs from the tubal angle to the ovary. The lateral wall of the uterus is connected with the lateral pelvic wall via the **Lig. latum uteri (12).** In the area of the cervix, the **Lig. sacrouterinum (14)** and the **Lig. cardinale (13)** connect the uterus with its adjacent organs.

Clinical remarks

With ovulation, the ovum is intercepted by the Infundibulum tubae uterinae and carried further in the Fallopian tube. Fertilisation of the ovum usually occurs in the Fallopian tube. **Inflammations of the Fallopian tube** can lead to its occlusion. Occlusions on both sides of the Fallopian tube lead to sterility. A partial occlusion of the tube can lead to dysfunction in the transport of the ovum and can cause an **ectopic pregnancy**.

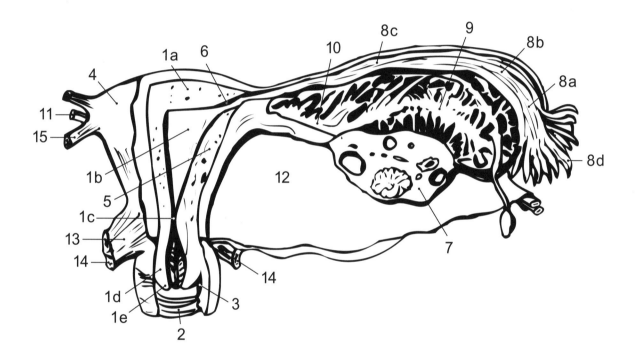

Abb. 6.10

135

7.1 Skull (cranium)

The bony skull, is comprised of:
- a **neurocranium (braincase)**
- a **viscerocranium (facial bones)**

The neurocranium consists of the calvaria (cranial roof) and the Basis cranii (cranial base). The cranial bones are connected to each other by cranial sutures (Suturae cranii). In the skull of the child, these sutures are represented by cartilaginous or fascial connections, which eventually fuse as synostoses.

Lateral view   In this view, the following structures which form the calvaria are distinguishable:
- the **Os frontale (1)**
- the **Os parietale (2, paired)**
- the **Squama occipitalis** of the **Os occipitale (3)**
- the **Pars squamosa (4a)** of the **Os temporale (4, paired)**

In the lateral view, the greater wing (ala major) of the sphenoid bone **(5, paired)** can be seen.
The following important cranial sutures of the cranial roof can be seen:
- The **Sutura coronalis (coronal suture, 6)** connects the Os frontale and the Ossa parietalia.
- The **Sutura lambdoidea (lambdoid suture, 7)** connects the Os occipitale and the Ossa parietalia.

In the side view of the Os temporale, the **Pars squamosa (4a)** as well as the **Pars petrosa (4b)** and the **Pars tympanica (4c)** can be seen: these three bony parts confine the **Porus acusticus externus (8)**.
The further occipitally located **Processus mastoideus (4d)** of the Pars petrosa contains the pneumatic Cellulae mastoideae, which are connected to the middle ear. Below the Porus acusticus externus lies the **Processus styloideus (4e)**, from where suprahyoid muscles originate.
The **Fossa mandibularis (socket of the mandibular joint, 4f)** lies immediately in front of the **Porus acusticus externus (8)** in the Pars squamosa of the Os temporale (4a). The Fossa mandibularis forms the mandibular joint with the **Processus condylaris (9a)** of the **mandibula (9)**. The further rostrally located **Processus coronoideus (9b)** of the mandibula serves as the insertion point for the masticatory muscles.

Frontal view   In this view, the **viscerocranium** can be seen, consisting of the following bones:
- **maxilla (10, paired)**

- **Os lacrimale (11, paired)**
- **Os nasale (12, paired)**
- **Os zygomaticum (13, paired)**
- **Os ethmoidale (14)**
- **Vomer (15)**
- **Conchae nasales inferiores (16)**
- **Os palatinum (paired,** not shown)
- **Mandibula (9)**

The body of the **maxilla (10)** contains the pneumatic maxillary sinus. The Processus alveolaris maxillae are the tooth-bearing bones of the upper jaw or maxilla. The maxilla forms a part of the bony confinement of the orbita (eye socket). The Os zygomaticum forms the prominent cheekbones and connects with the **Os temporale (4)** via the arch of the zygomatic bone.
The bony skeleton of the **nose** consists of the **Ossa nasalia (12)** and the **maxilla (10)**. The bony **nasal septum** is partially formed by the Lamina perpendicularis of the **Os ethmoidale (14)** and partially by the **vomer (15)**. Just like the upper nasal concha (not shown), the middle nasal concha, visible in the nasal cavity, belongs to the Os ethmoidale (14), while the **Conchae nasales inferiores (16)** display distinct bones.
Above the orbita in the Os frontale, and below the orbita in the maxilla, the **Foramen infraorbitale (18)** can be discerned on both sides of the **Foramen supraorbitale (17)**.
The **mandibula (9)** contains the teeth of the lower jaw and continues dorsally via the Angulus mandibulae into the Processus condylaris (9a) and into the Processus coronoideus (9b). The **Foramen mentale (19)** can be seen in the area of the chin.

> **Note**
>
> The Foramen supraorbitale, the Foramen infraorbitale and the Foramen mentale are the **nerve exit points for the three terminal branches of the N. trigeminus:**
> - **N. ophthalmicus (N. V/1)**
> - **N. maxillaris (N. V/2)**
> - **N. mandibularis (N. V/3)**

Clinical remarks

When the terminal branches of the N. trigeminus are irritated (e.g. with **sinusitis**), pressure on these nerve exit points causes pain.

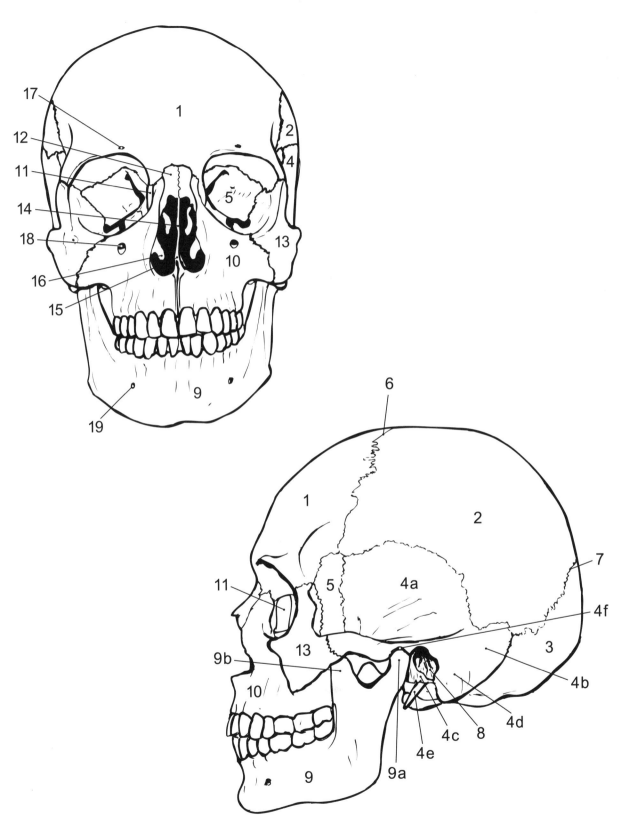

Abb. 7.1

7.2 Inner view of the base of the skull

The base of the skull consists of four unpaired bones, the
- **Os frontale (frontal bone, 1)**
- **Os ethmoidale (ethmoid bone, 2)**
- **Os sphenoidale (sphenoid bone, 3)**
- **Os occipitale (occipital bone, 4)**

as well as the paired
- **Os temporale (temporal bone, 5)**.

The inner base of the skull also shows three fossa arranged consecutively:
- the **anterior cranial fossa (Fossa cranii anterior, I)**, which accommodates the frontal lobes of the cerebrum
- the **middle cranial fossa (Fossa cranii media, II)**, wherein the temporal lobes of the cerebrum are located
- the **posterior cranial fossa (Fossa cranii posterior, III)**, which contains the cerebellum and parts of the brainstem

Anterior cranial fossa (I)　The **Lamina cribrosa (ethmoid bone plate, 2a)** of the Os ethmoidale (2) lies in the middle, punctured by numerous small holes for the Fila olfactoria (olfactory neural fibres) to pass through to the nasal cavity. On the Lamina cribrosa there is a raised ledge, the **Crista galli (2b)**, which serves as an insertion point for the Falx cerebri. Laterally of the Lamina cribrosa, on both sides, the Partes orbitales of the Os frontale (1) form the partition to the orbita lying below it. The **Corpus ossis sphenoidalis (3a)** and both the **Alae minores ossis sphenoidalis (lesser wing of the sphenoid bone, 3b)**, which join the **Processus clinoidei anteriores (3c)**, represent the border of the middle cranial fossa.

Middle cranial fossa (II)　The **Sella turcica (3d)** connects to this, bounded occipitally by the **Dorsum sellae (3e)**, and houses the pituitary gland. The **Canales optici (6)** lead to the orbita and serve as penetration points for the Nn. optici. Below the Alae minores ossis sphenoidalis (3b), the orbita is also reached from the middle cranial fossa via the **Fissura orbitalis superior (7)**. Here the cranial nerves, incl. the N. III, IV, V/1 and VI, pass through into the orbita. In the **ala major (3f)** of the Os sphenoidale, the Sella turcica is visible laterally and the **petrous pyramid (Pars petrosa ossis temporalis, 3g)**, the **Foramen rotundum (8)**, the **Foramen ovale (9)** and the **Foramen spinosum (10)** rostrally of the apex. They represent the openings for the second and third branch of the N. trigeminus (N. maxillaris: Foramen rotundum; N. mandibularis: Foramen ovale) and/or for the A. meningea media (Foramen spinosum).

On a skull which has not been macerated, the **Foramen lacerum (11)** is closed with a cartilaginous sheet. Here the N. petrosus major and the N. petrosus profundus pass through. Directly behind the Foramen lacerum lies the inner opening of the **Canalis caroticus (12)**, through which the A. carotis interna enters intracranially.

Posterior cranial fossa (III)　The posterior cranial fossa commences behind and below the Dorsum sellae and the edge of the petrous pyramid. Amongst others, parts of the brainstem and the Aa. vertebrales pass through the **Foramen magnum (13)** . The Aa. vertebrales unite intracranially with the A. basilaris on the **clivus (14)**. The **Sulcus sinus transversi (15)** and the **Sulcus sinus sigmoidei (16)** are located in the posterior cranial fossa. These recesses are caused by the eponymous venous sinus of the dura mater. The Sulcus sinus sigmoidei runs towards the **Foramen jugulare (17)**. Here the Sinus sigmoideus empties into the V. jugularis interna. Above the Foramen jugulare is the **Porus acusticus internus (18)**, through which the Nn. facialis and vestibulocochlearis penetrate into the petrous pyramid.

Clinical remarks

Because the skull base contains numerous openings for nerves and blood vessels, these structures are vulnerable following a **basal skull fracture**: on the one hand it can lead to **intracranial bleeding** from venous sinuses of the dura mater or from the meningeal arteries, and on the other hand nerve lesions lead, according to the affected nerve, to a characteristic **paralysis, sensory impairment** or **other malfunction symptoms**. In this way, fractures of the petrous pyramid involving an injury to the inner ear can lead to **hearing loss and vertigo.**

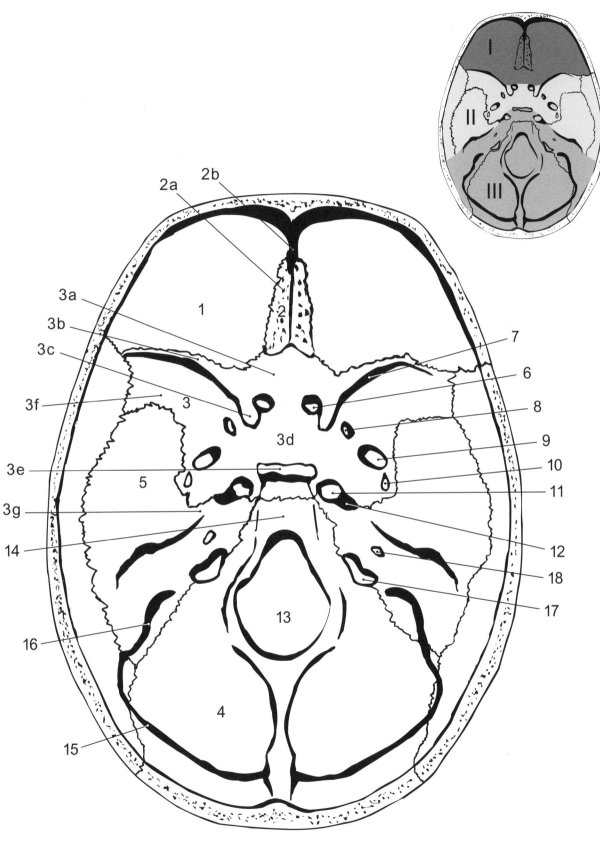

Abb. 7.2

7.3 Exterior view of the base of the skull

The outer base of the skull becomes visible after removal of the mandibula. The anterior third of the outer base of the skull is related to the viscerocranium, the posterior two-thirds of the neurocranium (➤ Chap. 7.1).

The hard palate consists rostrally of the paired **Proc. palatinus of the maxilla (1).** Both the Processus palatini include the **Foramen incisivum (2)** in the median. The edge of the posterior hard palate abuts the likewise paired **Lamina horizontalis of the Os palatinum (3),** penetrated by the **Foramen palatinum majus (4)**.

Where it joins the edge of the palate, the dorsal entrance to the nasal cavity is shown, the **choanae (opening to the nasal cavity, 5)**. Between the choanae, the **vomer (6)** forms the posterior part of the bony nasal septum.

From the body of the **Os sphenoidale (7)** going outwards, the **alae majore (greater wings of the sphenoid bone, 8)** expand laterally to both sides. The **Foramen ovale (9)** and the **Foramen spinosum (10)** can be discerned at the base of the ala major. The third branch of the N. trigeminus (N. mandibularis) passes through the Foramen ovale and the A. meningea media passes through the Foramen spinosum.

The Processus pterygoideus with the **Lamina lateralis (11)** and the **Lamina medialis (12)** originates from down below on both sides of the Os sphenoidale. The Lamina lateralis (11) serves the M. pterygoideus lateralis as an insertion point. The M. pterygoideus medialis arises in the fossa (Fossa pterygoidea) between both the laminae. The Lamina medialis (12) terminates in the **Hamulus pterygoideus (13)**.

The **Canalis caroticus (15)** lies in the **Os temporale (14)**, through which the A. carotis interna passes into the skull. Laterally thereof is the **Proc. styloideus (16)**, which is a point of origin for some of the suprahyoid muscles. Directly behind the base of the Processus styloideus, the **Foramen stylomastoideum (17)** can be seen, the exit point of the N. facialis. The **Proc. mastoideus (18)** also belongs to the Os temporale with the **Foramen mastoideum (19)** lying behind it. In front of the **Porus acusticus externus (20),** the **Fossa mandibularis (21)** forms the socket of the mandibular joint.

In the occipital area of the skull base, the posterior edge of the Pars basalis of the Os temporale (14), together with the **Os occipitale (22),** borders the **Foramen jugulare (23),** which is surrounded by the Fossa jugularis, where the V. jugularis interna begins.

The **Foramen magnum (24)** proceeds through the Os occipitale (22), linking the intracranial area with the vertebral canal. The Foramen magnum serves, amongst others, as an opening for parts of the brainstem and/or for the Aa. vertebrales. Rostrally of the Foramen magnum, the **Tuberculum pharyngeum (25)** lies on the Pars basalis of the Os occipitale and serves the pharyngeal muscles as an insertion point. Laterally of the Foramen magnum, the **Condyli occipitales (26)** can be seen, two biconvex articular processes, which form the upper cranial joint, along with the upper cervical vertebra (atlas).

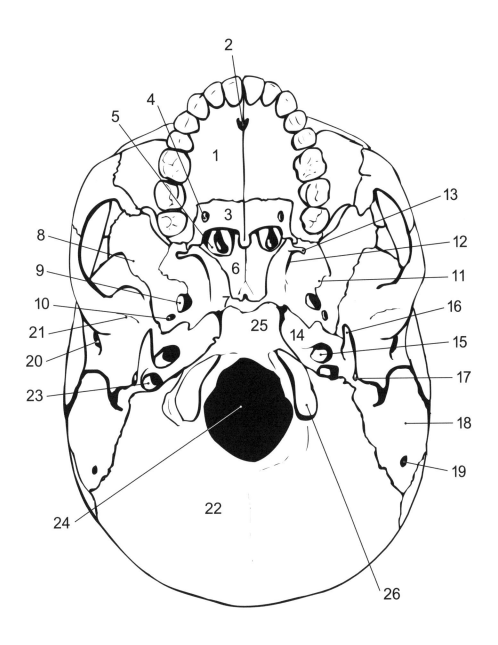

Abb. 7.3

141

7.4 Mimetic muscles

The mimetic muscles are striated and lie in the head and neck area in the subcutaneous fatty tissue. They contain no fascia and insert directly into the skin. This facilitates fine facial movements, essential for facial expression. The mimetic muscles are innervated by the terminal motor branches of the N. facialis (N. VII).

Forehead area   The **M. epicranius (1)** extends from the back of the head to the forehead area. It is subdivided by the **Galea aponeurotica (2)** into a Venter frontalis and a Venter occipitalis (not shown). The M. epicranius enables frowning.

Eye area   With the **M. orbicularis oculi (3),** a Pars orbitalis at the edge of the orbita and a Pars palpebralis, which covers the lids, can be seen. The fibres of the muscles encircle the eye. They facilitate blinking as well as squeezing the eyes shut.
The **M. corrugator supercilii (4)** runs from the bridge of the nose ascending to lateral to the middle of the eyebrow. It places the skin over the bridge of the nose in perpendicular folds.

Mouth and cheek area   The fibres of the **M. orbicularis oris (5)** encircle the mouth. Some of the fibres (Pars labialis) form the muscle parts of the lips. With respective tensing of the various muscle parts, the lips can be tightly closed, partly opened or pursed.
The **M. depressor labii inferioris (6)** originates from the mandibula and inserts into the lower lip. It pulls down the lower lip. Medially to the M. depressor labii inferioris, the **M. mentalis (7)** runs from the alveoli of the lower incisors to the dimple in the chin. Its fibres pull the skin on the chin upwards, thereby creating a groove between the chin and the lower lip. The **M. depressor anguli oris (8)** adjoins laterally of the M. depressor labii inferioris. Its fibres insert in the area of the corner of the mouth in the M. orbicularis oris and facilitate the pulling down of the corners of the mouth.
The fibres of the **M. risorius (9)** extend from the skin on the cheeks to the corners of the mouth. They retract the angle of the mouth widely and create dimples in the cheeks. The **Mm. zygomatici major (10)** and **minor (11)** originate on the arch of the zygomatic bone and run across the cheeks to the corners of the mouth and/or the upper lip. They are typically used during smiling/laughing, facilitating a happy facial expression.
The **M. levator labii superioris alaeque nasi (12)** lies medially of these muscles. It runs from the Margo infraorbitalis to the upper lip and lifts them as well as the nostrils. The **M. levator anguli oris (13)** runs from the Foramen infraorbitale to the corners of the mouth and pulls these upwards.

The **M. nasalis (14)** lies on and next to the nasal skeleton. Its Pars transversa lifts the upper lip and induces a groove between the nose and the mouth. The Pars alaris inserts on both sides in the dorsal aponeurosis of the nose and can pull down the cartilaginous part of the nose. After removing the superficial layer of the mimetic muscles, the **M. buccinator (15)** on the cheeks becomes visible. It forms the muscular base of the cheeks, stretches when blowing up the cheeks with air and can then, along with the M. orbicularis oris, blow it out again. With a one-sided action it pulls down the corner of the mouth on the same side. When chewing, it can push food which has moved in between the row of teeth and the cheek back into the oral cavity.
In the illustration, the **Gl. parotis (parotid gland, 16)** with its **deferent duct**, the **Ductus parotideus (17)**, also becomes visible on the left side of the head after dissecting the superficial layer of the mimetic muscles. The Ductus parotideus crosses over the **M. masseter ([18]**; this belongs to the masticatory muscles and is innervated by the branches from the N. mandibularis) as well as the buccal fat pad, and finally penetrates the M. buccinator to empty in the Vestibulum oris across from the 2nd upper molars.

Neck area   The mimetic muscles extend in the form of **platysma muscles (19)** across the neck to the clavicle. By tensing the platysma muscle strongly, its muscle fibres become visible through the skin as longitudinal folds.

Note

The mimetic muscles are striated and without fascia. They lie in the subcutaneous fatty tissue of the head and neck and are innervated by the terminal motor branches of the N. facialis.

Clinical remarks

For a clinical **nerve function test of the N. facialis (N. VII),** the patient is asked to frown, to close the eyes tightly, to bare the teeth and to purse the lips as if to whistle. With **peripheral facial nerve paralysis** all mimetic muscles on the affected side fail, but with **central facial nerve paralysis** frowning and blinking are still possible.

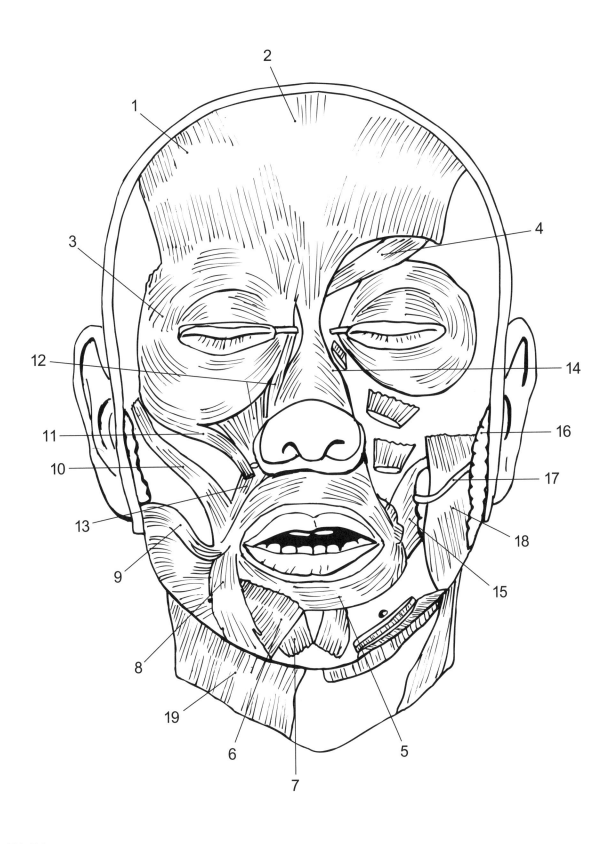

Abb. 7.4

7.5 Mandibular joint and masticatory muscles

Mandibular joint   The mandibular joint becomes visible after removing the Os zygomaticum.

The mandibular joint is a gliding hinge joint: it enables the opening and closing of the mouth as well as the grinding and sliding movements of the lower jaw.

The mandibular joint consists of the following parts:

- Fossa mandibularis
- Discus articularis
- Caput mandibulae

The socket of the mandibular joint is formed by the **Fossa mandibularis (1)** of the **Os temporale (2)**. It is bounded rostrally by a slight raise, the Tuberculum articulare (not shown). The socket articulates around the cartilaginous **Discus articularis (3)** with the **caput (4)** of the **mandibula (5)**.

The Discus articularis facilitates congruence between the joint surfaces. It is movable and can increase the joint surface rostrally with grinding and sliding movements.

The mandibular joint contains a joint capsule where the masticatory muscles (see below) insert.

Masticatory muscles   The masticatory muscles consist of the following muscles:

- M. pterygoideus medialis
- M. pterygoideus lateralis
- M. masseter
- M. temporalis

The **M. pterygoideus medialis (6)** originates in the Fossa pterygoidea of the Os sphenoidale (not shown), runs downwards and inserts on the inside of the **Angulus mandibulae (7)** on the Tuberositas pterygoidea. There it is connected tendinously to the M. masseter which inserts on the outside, so that a loop of muscle is formed around the Corpus mandibulae.

The **M. pterygoideus lateralis (8)** originates bicephalically on the Lamina lateralis of the Processus pterygoideus and on the Crista infratemporalis of the ala major of the Os sphenoidale (not shown). It runs almost horizontally to the back, to the **Collum mandibulae (9)** as well as to the **Discus articularis (3)**, and to the joint capsule of the mandibular joint.

The **M. masseter (10)** originates from the bottom edge of the **zygomatic arch (Arcus zygomaticus, 11)**, runs downwards and inserts on the outside of the Corpus mandibulae up to the **Processus coronoideus (12)**.

The **M. temporalis (13)** originates with a broad base on the Squama ossis temporalis, runs medially of the zygomatic arch downwards and inserts on the Processus coronoideus.

The masticatory muscles are innervated by the short branches of the N. mandibularis (N. V/3) from its 'Portio minor' (➤ Chap. 7.6).

Masticatory movement   The mouth is opened with the muscles of the floor of the mouth and supported by the M. pterygoideus lateralis. The M. temporalis and the muscle loop of the M. masseter and the M. pterygoideus medialis are mostly responsible for closing the mouth and biting.

With grinding and sliding movements in the mandibular joint, the different parts of the four masticatory muscles work together in different configurations. Especially the M. pterygoideus lateralis with its horizontal pathway is able to move the mandibula rostrally. Thereby the Discus articularis is also pulled forwards which enlarges the joint socket.

Clinical remarks

In many patients, extreme mouth opening can lead to a **dislocation of the Caput mandibulae**. Herein the joint head moves forwards out of the joint socket and gets caught in front of the Tuberculum mandibulae. The result is a painful **lockjaw**. To reset the jaw, the mandibula is first moved downwards past the Tuberculum articulare and only then backwards into the joint socket.

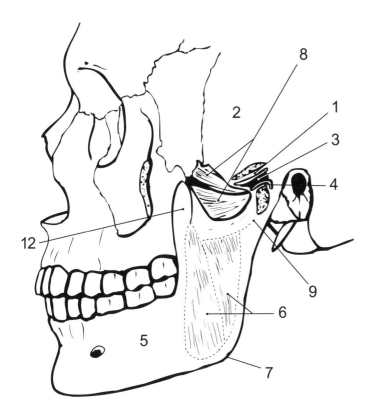

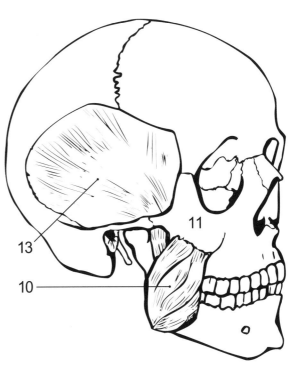

Abb. 7.5

7.6 Deep facial area

The deep facial area is exposed after removing the mimetic muscle, the M. masseter, the zygomatic arch as well as the Processus condylaris and coronoideus. This extends on both sides laterally of the zygomatic arch and from the mandibular branches medially to the pharynx and to the Processus pterygoideus of the Os sphenoidale.

The deep facial area is largely filled out by the **M. pterygoideus lateralis (1)** and by the **M. pterygoideus medialis (2)**. In between these are the bifurcation areas of the A. maxillaris and of the N. mandibularis.

The **A. maxillaris (3)** branches off as a terminal branch of the **A. carotis externa (4)** behind the Collum mandibulae. The second large terminal branch of the A. carotis externa, the **A. temporalis superficialis (5)**, runs together with the **N. auriculotemporalis (6)** upwards in front of the ear, to branch out superficially in the temporal area (➤ Chap. 7.10).

In the deep facial area, the A. maxillaris branches off into its terminal branches, of which the following can be seen:

* A. alveolaris inferior
* A. buccalis
* A. temporalis profunda
* A. infraorbitalis

The terminal branches of the A. maxillaris are accompanied by the eponymous terminal branches of the N. mandibularis (not shown).

The **A. alveolaris inferior (7)** runs together with the eponymous **N. alveolaris inferior (8)** in the (opened here) **Canalis alveolaris** of the mandibula. Before passing into the canal, the N. alveolaris inferior provides the **N. mylohyoideus (9)**, which proceeds into the Trigonum submandibulare and innervates some of the muscles of the floor of the mouth.

The **A. buccalis (10)** proceeds together with the **N. buccalis (11)** to the **M. buccinator (12)**. There the A. buccalis anastomoses with the branches of the A. facialis, which originate from the A. carotis externa (not shown).

The branches of the **A. temporalis profunda,** the Aa. temporales **profundae anterior (13a)** and **posterior (13b),** branch out with the accompanying **Nn. temporales profundi anterior (14a)** and **posterior (14b)** into the deep parts of the **M. temporalis (15)**.

In the area of the **Foramen infraorbitale (18)**, the **A. infraorbitalis (16)** moves together with the **N. infraorbitalis (17)** to the surface. In the Canalis infraorbitalis, branches bifurcate from the A. infraorbitalis to the teeth and to the gums of the upper jaw. As a terminal branch of the N. mandibularis, the

N. lingualis (19) appears between the Mm. pterygoidei medialis and lateralis and then descends in the direction of the Trigonum submandibulare. The **Chorda tympani**, which contains preganglionic parasympathetic fibres and taste fibres from the N. intermedius (not shown), adjoins the N. lingualis.

As with all the mimetic muscles, the **M. buccinator** is innervated by the **N. facialis** and not, for instance, by the N. buccalis from the N. mandibularis, which provide sensory innervation to the skin and mucosa of the cheeks.

The **N. mandibularis** is the third branch of the important **sensory** cranial nerve, the N. trigeminus. Additionally the N. mandibularis contains **specific visceroefferent** fibres of the so-called **Portio minor**, which innervates the masticatory muscles and, via the N. mylohyoideus, some of the muscles of the floor of the mouth with short branches.

Along its pathway, the **Chorda tympani** is taken up by the sensory N. lingualis. Its parasympathetic fibres however originate from the **N. intermedius** (a part of the N. facialis).

The **N. alveolaris inferior** can be anaesthetized from the oral cavity, before its point of entry into the Foramen mandibulae with so-called conductive anaesthesia. This ensures a painfree procedure to the teeth of the lower jaw.

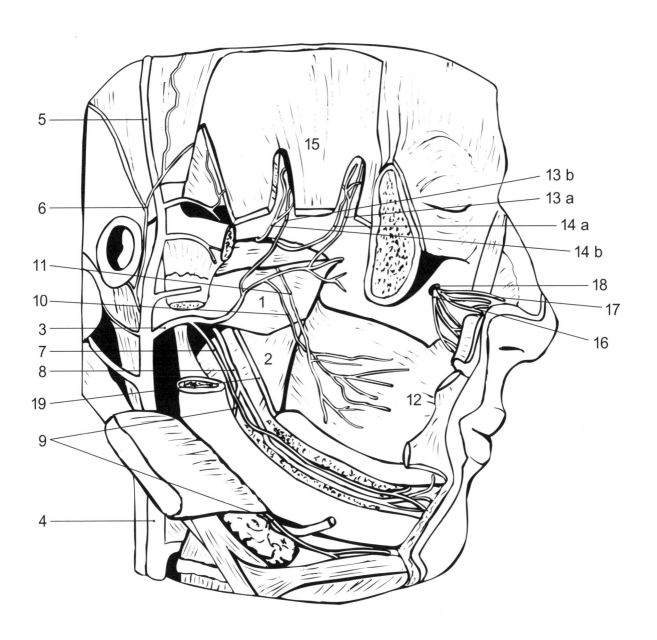

5

6

11

10

3

7

8

19

9

4

15

13 b

13 a

14 a

14 b

18

17

16

1

2

12

Abb. 7.6

147

7.7 Orbit and extrinsic eye muscles

Orbita The orbit (eye socket) has the shape of a four-sided pyramid, with the base pointing rostrally and the apex occipitally. The illustration above shows the right orbita.
The orbita consists of the following bones:

- **Os frontale (1a and b)**
- **Os zygomaticum (2a–c)**
- **Maxilla (3a and b)**
- **Os lacrimale (4)**
- **Os ethmoidale (5)**
- **Os palatinum (6)**
- **Os sphenoidale (7a and b)**

Boundaries of the orbita The **orbital entrance (Aditus orbitalis)** is bounded supraorbitally by the **Os frontale (1a)**, laterally below by the **Os zygomaticum (2a)** and infraorbitally by the **maxilla (3a)**.
The **nasal orbital wall** consists of the **Os lacrimale (4)**, which shows a conspicuous bulge for the lacrimal sac, and the **Lamina orbitalis of the Os ethmoidale (5)**. Through its thin bony wall, the pneumatic spaces of the Os ethmoidale (Cellulae ethmoidales) show through on the skull.
The **orbital floor** is formed by the **Os zygomaticum (2b),** by the **maxilla (3b)** and by the **Processus orbitalis of the Os palatinum (6)**. If the Sinus maxillaris is enlarged, the floor of the orbita in this area of the maxilla can be very thin.
The **temporal orbital wall** consists of the Facies orbitalis of the Os zygomaticum (2c) and the **ala major of the Os sphenoidale (7a)**.
The **orbital roof** consists of the **Facies orbitalis of the Os frontale (1b)** and the **ala minor of the Os sphenoidale (7b)**.
The **Fissura orbitalis inferior (8)** divides the temporal wall from the floor of the orbita. The **Fissura orbitalis superior (9)** lies between the roof and temporal wall and serves amongst others as an opening for the Nn. oculomotorius, trochlearis, abducens and for the V. ophthalmica.
The N. opticus and the A. ophthalmica pass through the **Canalis nervi optici (10)** into the orbita.

Eye muscles The six striated outer eye muscles move the **Bulbus oculi (11)** and thereby enable a change in the line of sight. The illustration below shows the eye muscle of the right eyeball from above. The following eye muscles can be seen:

- **four rectus eye muscles** (M. rectus superior, M. rectus inferior, M. rectus lateralis and M. rectus medialis)
- **two oblique eye muscles** (M. obliquus superior and M. obliquus inferior)

The four rectus eye muscles, **M. rectus superior (12)**, **M. rectus inferior (13)**, **M. rectus lateralis (14)** and **M. rectus medialis (15)**, originate in the depths of the orbita in the area of the Canalis nervi optici (10). They run rostrally and insert into the sclera of the Bulbus oculi. According to their pathway, they turn the eyeball upwards, downwards, temporally or nasally.
The M. rectus lateralis is innervated by the N. abducens, and all other straight eye muscles are innervated by the N. oculomotorius.
The **M. obliquus superior (16)** originates along with the straight eye muscles in the area of the Canalis nervi optici (10) and then proceeds rostrally via the M. rectus medialis on the nasal wall of the orbita. There its direction of movement is turned around in a tendinous loop, the **trochlea (17)**, and it inserts obliquely towards the back into the upper side of the eyeball. It is innervated by the N. trochlearis and facilitates a lowering of the line of sight as well as an internal rotation and abduction of the eyeball.
The **M. obliquus inferior (18)** originates as a single eye muscle from the floor of the orbita and encompasses the eyeball obliquely from below. It is innervated by the N. oculomotorius and leads to a raising of the line of sight as well as an external rotation and abduction of the eyeball.

Note

Eye muscle	Innervation	Line of sight
M. obliquus superior	N. trochlearis (N. IV)	downwards temporal
M. rectus lateralis	N. abducens (N. VI)	temporal
M. rectus superior	N. oculomotorius (N. III)	upwards
M. rectus inferior	N. oculomotorius (N. III)	downwards
M. rectus medialis	N. oculomotorius (N. III)	nasal
M. obliquus inferior	N. oculomotorius (N. III)	upwards temporal

Clinical remarks

With **paralysis of an outer eye muscle,** the eyeball deviates from the central position in the direction of the antagonist of the paralysed muscle. The patient typically complains of **double vision.** This double vision increases when trying to turn the line of sight to the direction of movement of the paralysed muscle.

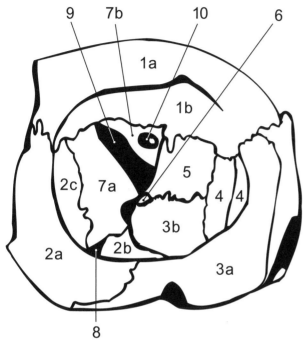

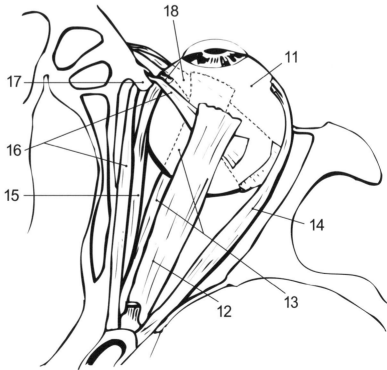

Abb. 7.7

7.8 Horizontal section through the right Bulbus oculi

The **cornea (1)** is the first structure present when following the optical path of a beam of light into the eye. It is transparent, convex towards the front, and with its fixed refractive power contributes to the total refractive power of the eye. The cornea does not contain blood vessels but is fed via diffusion.

Behind the cornea lies the **anterior eye chamber (2)**, filled with intraocular fluid. The intraocular fluid is formed in the **posterior eye chamber (3)** in the area of the **Corpus ciliare (4)**, passes through the **pupil (6)**, which is bounded by the **iris (5)**, into the anterior chamber and is there reabsorbed in the **Schlemm's canal (7)**.

The **iris (5)** contains the Mm. sphincter and dilatator pupillae. The **M. sphincter pupillae (8)** runs circularly on the inner edge of the iris and constricts the pupil. The **M. dilatator pupillae (9)** has a radial fibre course and thereby dilates the pupil.

The back of the iris is adjacent to the **lens (10)** in the area of the pupil. The lens is transparent and biconvex. It enables accommodation (i.e. it changes the refractive power of the eye depending on the distance of the fixed object). The lens is suspended via **zonular fibres (11)** in the **Corpus ciliare (4)**. The traction of the zonular fibres holds the lens in a flattened state, with less refractive power. If the M. ciliaris, situated in the Corpus ciliare, contracts, the ciliary muscle moves itself forward and the zonular fibres relax. Thereby the lens can return to its more spherical resting position, and its refractive power increases (near-point accommodation).

The **Corpus vitreum (vitreous body, 12)** adjoins the lens dorsally. It occupies most of the Bulbus oculi and consists of a transparent, watery, gelatinous mass.

The **retina (13)** lies directly on the Corpus vitreum. The point of clearest vision, the **Fovea centralis (14)**, lies in the centre of the optical axis and is characterised by its particularly closely juxtaposed photoreceptors. Nasally of the Fovea centralis, the **N. opticus (15)** passes into the Bulbus oculi. The **Discus nervi optici (16)** is found at the point at which it reaches the retina. It is also described as the blind spot, as there are no photoreceptors in this area.

On the outside, the **choroidea (17)** adjoins the retina. In it, the branches of the A. und V. ophthalmica supply the eye.

The outer layer of the Bulbus oculi form the **sclera (18)**. The **outer eye muscles (19)**, which move the eyeball, insert into it.

Note

The **M. sphincter pupillae** is parasympathetically innervated via the N. oculomotorius and constricts the pupil.
The **M. dilatator pupillae** is sympathetically innervated from the cervical ganglia of the sympathetic trunk and dilates the pupil.

Clinical remarks

With **shortsightedness (myopia),** the axial length of the Bulbus oculi is too long in comparison with its refractive power. Rays of light focus in front of, instead of on, the retina, resulting in blurred vision.
With **farsightedness (hyperopia),** the axial length of the Bulbus oculi is too short. This also results in blurred vision, as the broken rays of light only focus behind the retina.

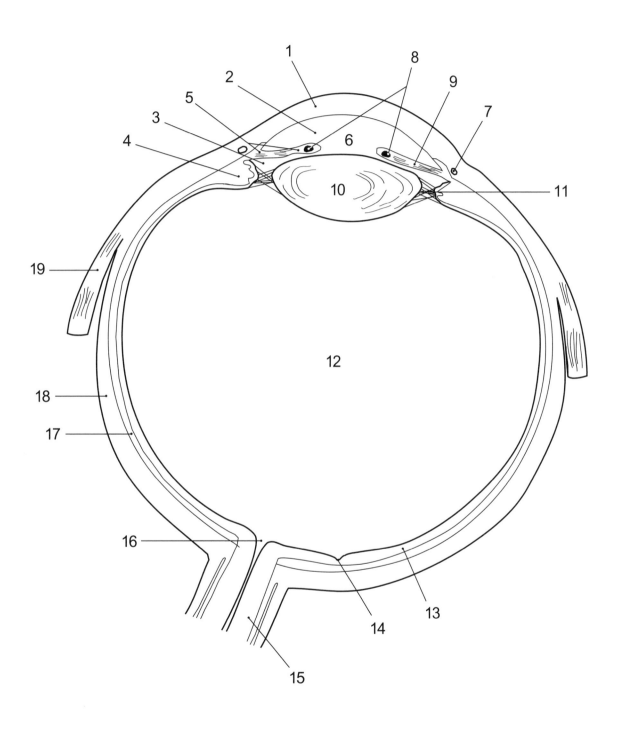

Abb. 7.8

7.9 Auditory canals and the middle ear

The hearing and vestibular organ is a complex structure located in the Pars petrosa of the **Os temporale (1)**. The depiction shows an oblique section through the **outer auditory canal (Meatus acusticus externus)**, the **middle ear (Auris media)** and the **inner auditory canal (Meatus acusticus internus)**.

Outer auditory canal (I)   The outer auditory canal starts cartilaginously at the external ear and passes into the Os temporale in the area of the Porus acusticus externus. It runs in a slightly S-shaped curve from cranial, lateral and occipital to caudal, medial and rostral. The outer auditory canal ends with the **Membrana tympani (eardrum, 2)**. The thin, transparent Membrana tympani forms the border between the external ear and the tympanic cavity. The Membrana tympani is oval and tapers down the middle into a funnel shape to the umbo. The umbo is formed by the manubrium (handle of the malleus), inserting on the tympanic side on the eardrum.

Middle ear (II)   The middle ear contains the three small auditory ossicles (Ossicula auditus):
- **malleus (3)**
- **incus (4)**
- **stapes (5)**

The **malleus (3),** partially removed here, is first in line on the chain of auditory bones. Adjoining it is the **incus (4)**, which has also been exposed down to its Proc. lenticularis. The incus is connected to the **stapes (5)**.
The auditory ossicles are connected articulately and transfer the vibrations of the eardrum, which are caused by sound waves, to the inner ear which is filled with perilymph. The stapes insert there at the **Fenestra vestibuli (oval window, 6)**.
The tympanic cavity is covered with mucosa and is connected to the **pneumatic cells of the Proc. mastoideus (7)**.
The **Chorda tympani (8)** runs through the tympanic cavity between the malleus and the incus. This branch of the N. intermedius contains gustatory fibres and preganglionic parasympathetic fibres. It reaches the outer base of the skull via the Fissura petrotympanica.
The **N. facialis (N. VII, 9)** runs in the Canalis nervi facialis, separated only by a thin bony wall from the middle ear.

Inner ear (III)   The inner ear is functionally divided into the hearing and vestibular organ. The illustration basically shows the section through the hearing organ, which lies in the cochlea.

The **cochlea (10)**, which consists of bone, has two and a half turns. Inside it there are three different cavities:
- Scala vestibuli
- Scala tympani
- Ductus cochlearis

The **Scala vestibuli (11)** and the **Scala tympani (12)** begin at the **oval window** (Fenestra vestibuli) and/or at the **Vestibulum (13)**. The Scala vestibuli ascends in a spiral to the apex of the cochlea. There it connects with the Scala tympani at the so-called helicotrema. This spirals to the base of the cochlea again and ends at the Fenestra cochleae (round window, not shown), which borders the tympanic cavity.
The **Ductus cochlearis (14)** is between the Scala tympani and the Scala vestibuli, which are both filled with perilymph. It is filled with endolymph and contains the sensory cells (hair cells), which sense the vibrations of the perilymph and thereby acoustic signals can be perceived.
The signals of the sensory cells are conducted via the **N. cochlearis (15)** to the brain. The N. cochlearis joins with the **N. vestibularis (16)** of the vestibular organ and runs as the **N. vestibulocochlearis (N. VIII, 17)** into the **Meatus acusticus internus (18)**.
Of the vestibular organ in this section, it is only possible to see parts of the **posterior semicircular canal (19)**.

Clinical remarks

In healthy individiuals, the eardrum has a pearly color, is transparent and is shaped like a funnel. With an otoscopy, a light reflex is thereby typically created in the anterior lower quadrant of the eardrum. **Changes in color and disappearance of the light reflex** indicate a disorder of the ear drum and/or the middle ear.
Inflammation can occur in the middle ear which is lined with mucosa, especially in children, when Cellulae mastoideae can be involved. Due to the anatomical proximity, it can not only lead to disturbed **sound conduction and pain,** but can also spread to the **structures of the middle cranial fossa** in the case of longer-lasting infections.

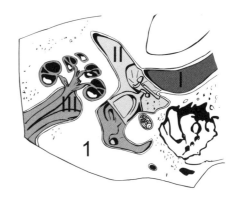

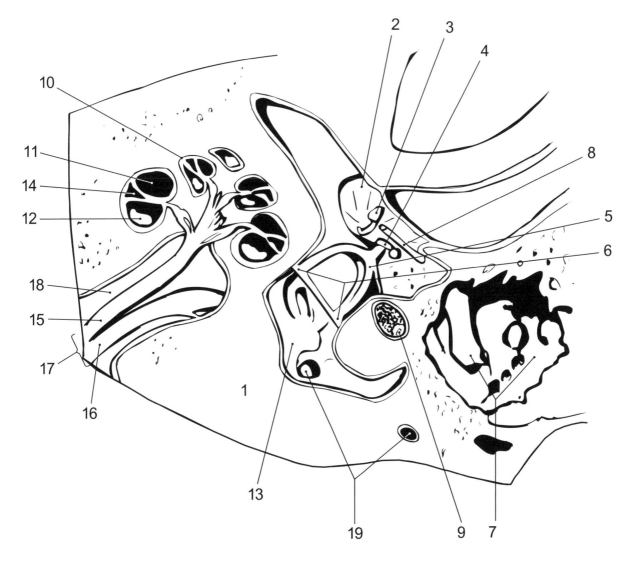

Abb. 7.9

153

7.10 Arteries of the head

The **A. carotis communis (1)** divides into the A. carotis externa and the A. carotis interna in the neck at the level of the thyroid cartilage.

While the **A. carotis interna (2)** proceeds to the base of the skull without any further branching out, the **A. carotis externa (3)** provides the following branches in the neck and the head:

- The **A. thyroidea superior (4)** branches first and runs in an arch-shape to caudal along the upper edge of the thyroid.
- The **A. lingualis (5)** is not shown. It turns to rostral and reaches the area of the floor of the mouth. It supplies the tongue, parts of the oral cavity and the floor of the mouth.
- The **A. facialis (6)** runs to rostral below the Glandula submandibularis (not shown) and turns at the anterior edge of the M. masseter around the rim of the mandibula. There its pulse can be palpated. It supplies the face. Its terminal branch, the **A. angularis (7)**, anastomoses in the area of the medial corner of the eye with the A. ophthalmica from the A. carotis interna (not shown).
- The small **A. pharyngea ascendens (8)** has not been shown. It ascends in the lateral wall of the pharynx. One of its terminal branches, the A. meningea posterior, passes through the Foramen jugulare to intracranial and there supplies parts of the dura mater.
- The **A. occipitalis (9)** runs underneath the posterior belly of the M. digastricus (not shown) to occipital and then turns cranially. To the side of the M. trapezius it again reaches the surface occipitally and branches off there into its terminal branches. The A. occipitalis supplies the back of the head and parts of the back of the neck.
- The **A. auricularis posterior (10)**, the most cranial outflow of the A. carotis externa, runs behind the external ear. It supplies parts of the external ear and the mastoid process, as well as parts of the middle ear and the Cellulae mastoideae (A. tympanica posterior).

The **A. temporalis superficialis (11)** and the **A. maxillaris (12)** are the terminal branches of the A. carotis externa:

- The **A. temporalis superficialis (11)** runs initially below the parotid gland and reaches the surface in front of the outer auditory canal. It provides the **A. transversa faciei (13)**, which runs below the arch of the zygomatic bone to the cheek and anastomoses there with branches of the A. facialis. On the forehead and in the temporal area, the A. temporalis superficialis branches off into its terminal branches.
- The **A. maxillaris (12)**, the largest terminal branch of the A. carotis externa, runs to rostral via the Fossa infratemporalis into the Fossa pterygopalatina. The A. maxillaris with its branches supplies, amongst others, the upper jaw, nasal cavities, gums, teeth, masticatory muscles and part of the dura mater.

The **A. alveolaris inferior (14)**, a large branch of the A. maxillaris, runs into the Canalis mandibulae. It supplies the lower jaw including the teeth and gums and reaches the bone surface once again via the Foramen mentale, as the R. mentalis.

The **A. infraorbitalis (15)**, a further bifurcation of the A. maxillaris, runs through the eponymous canal to the Foramen infraorbitale. Along its course, it supplies portions of the teeth, the gums and the mucosa of the upper jaw.

Next to the **A. carotis interna (2)**, the **Aa. vertebrales (16)** represent the second important inflow for the blood supply of the brain (➤ Chap. 9.6). They arise on both sides of the **A. subclavia (17)** and ascend in the Foramina transversaria of the 1st–6th cervical vertebrae, then passing into the Foramen magnum of the skull. There they unite on the clivus to the A. basilaris.

Note

The **order of the outflows of the A. carotis externa** can be memorised with the following mnemonic:
Some (A. thyroidea **s**uperior)
American (**A**. pharyngea ascendens)
ladies (A. **l**ingualis)
found (A. **f**acialis)
our (A. **o**ccipitalis)
pyramids (A. auricularis **p**osterior)
most (A. **m**axillaris).
satisfactory. (A. temporalis **s**uperficialis)

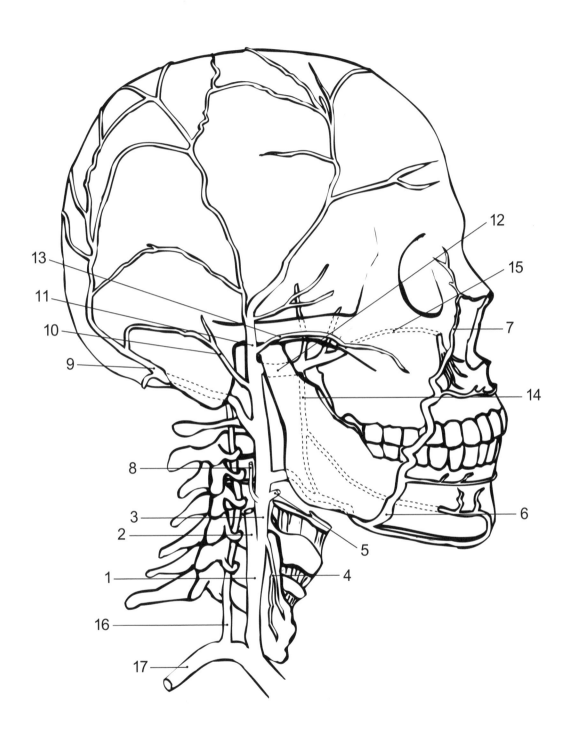

Abb. 7.10

7.11 Veins of the head

Vena jugularis interna The venous blood of the head and the brain are primarily drained via the **V. jugularis interna (1)**. It begins at the base of the skull at the Foramen jugulare, where it incorporates the blood from the venous sinuses of the brain. Further along its course, it runs alongside the N. vagus and the A. carotis in the carotid sheath of the neck and unites with the V. subclavia of the V. brachiocephalica (not shown) in the area of the sternoclavicular joint.

The **V. facialis (2),** which drains the venous blood from the facial area, empties in the V. jugularis interna.

The **V. angularis (3)** anastomoses with **terminal branches of the V. ophthalmica (4)** in the area of the medial corner of the eye and thereby connects with the intracranial venous sinuses (➤ Chap. 9.8).

- The **V. submentalis (5)** drains the chin area and the floor of the mouth and flows to the V. facialis.
- From the temporal and the skull area, the **V. temporalis superficialis (6)** flows to caudal into the **V. retromandibularis (7)**, which empties into the V. facialis or directly into the V. jugularis interna.

The **V. thyroidea superior (8)**, which comes from the thyroid, empties slightly below into the V. jugularis interna.

The **Plexus pterygoideus (9)** lies in the deep facial area between the Mm. pterygoidei. It has connections to the venous sinuses of the intracranial dura mater, to the V. facialis (2) or also directly to the V. jugularis interna (1).

The venous blood of the skullcap and the dura mater is drained by the **diploic veins (10)**. They are located in the spongy bone of the skull and can drain off either to the venous sinuses of the dura mater or via the so-called emissaries of the outer veins of the head.

Vena jugularis externa Coming from the back of the head, the **V. auricularis posterior (11)** and the **V. occipitalis (12)** unite with the **V. jugularis externa (13)**. These can connect to the drainage area of the V. jugularis interna via anastomoses with the V. retromandibularis. Contrary to this, it does however run superficially below the platysma on the neck to caudal and empties in the area of the upper thoracic aperture, either into the V. jugularis interna, the V. subclavia or into the V. brachiocephalica.

Note

The V. jugularis interna represents the main drainage route of the venous blood from the head and the brain. Venous valves are rare in the head and neck area, and **blood flow in both directions** is possible.

Clinical remarks

A connection is present between the extracranial drainage routes and the venous sinuses of the intracranial dura mater called the V. angularis (3). In some cases, pathogens can arrive **intracranially** via this route **from the lateral facial area** (e.g. with abscesses) where they can cause a thrombosis of the venous sinuses.

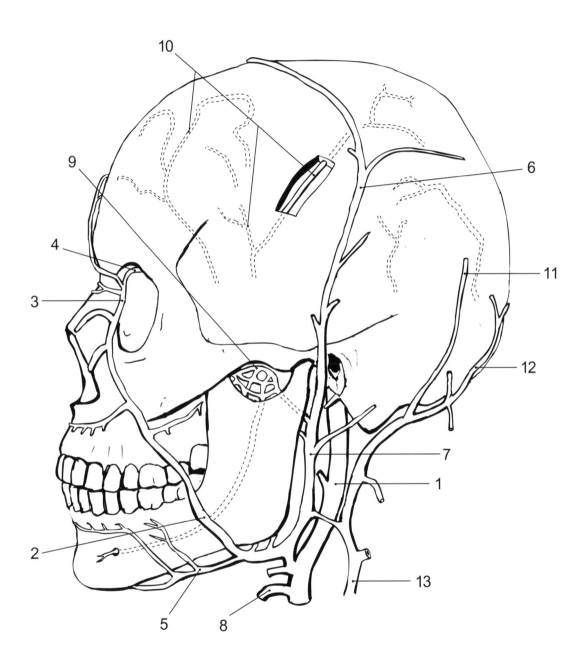

Abb. 7.11

157

8.1 Areas of the neck

Two large topographical areas can be demarcated in the neck:
- the **Regio cervicalis anterior (I)**
- the **Regio cervicalis lateralis (II)**

Regio cervicalis anterior (I) This area is confined by the lower rim of the **mandibula (1)**, the midline of the neck and the anterior edge of the **M. sternocleidomastoideus (2)**. Inside the Regio cervicalis anterior, further areas can be identified:
- the **Trigonum submandibulare (Ia)**
- the **Trigonum caroticum (Ib)**

The **Trigonum submandibulare (Ia)** is the area between the lower rim of the **mandibula (1)** and both the bellies of the **M. digastricus (3)**. Inside this triangle are situated amongst others the eponymous **Gl. submandibularis (submandibular gland, 4)**. The **muscles of the floor of the mouth (5)** delimit the Trigonum submandibulare up to the oral cavity.

The **Trigonum caroticum (Ib)** is situated between the lower rim of the Venter posterior of the **M. digastricus (3)**, the anterior edge of the **M. sternocleidomastoideus (2)** and the Venter superior of the **M. omohyoideus (6a)**. This area contains the A. carotis (and is named accordingly) which runs in the carotid sheath of the neck.

In the medial sections of the Regio cervicalis anterior are the superficial **infrahyoidal muscles (7)** and also in the depths, the visceral cord of the neck, which contains the **larynx (8)**, the **trachea (9)** and the **Gl. thyroidea (thyroid gland, 10)** as well as other entities.

Regio cervicalis lateralis (II) This area is confined by the posterior edge of the **M. sternocleidomastoideus (2)**, the upper edge of the **clavicula (11)** and by the **clavicula (12)**. The Venter inferior of the double-bellied **M. omohyoideus (6b)** subdivides the Regio cervicalis lateralis into:
- the **Trigonum omoclaviculare (Fossa supraclavicularis major, IIa)**
- the **Trigonum omotrapezoideum (IIb)**

M. omohyoideus and M. sternocleidomastoideus

The **M. omohyoideus (6)** belongs to the infrahyoid muscles. With its **Venter superior (6a)** it attaches to the **Os hyoideum (hyoid bone, 13)** and originates with its Venter inferior on the Margo superior of the scapula. Both the bellies are connected by an intermediate tendon.

The two-headed **M. sternocleidomastoideus (2)** originates on the sternum and clavicula and runs along the neck, ascending

to the Proc. mastoideus. With thin people it is possible to see the small **Fossa supraclavicularis minor (14)** between the two original heads.

Note

Area	Boundaries
Regio cervicalis anterior	lower edge of the mandibula, anterior edge of the M. sternocleidomastoideus
Trigonum submandibulare	lower edge of the mandibula, upper edge of the M. digastricus (Venter anterior and posterior)
Trigonum caroticum	lower edge of the M. digastricus (Venter posterior), upper edge of the M. omohyoideus (Venter superior), anterior edge of the M. sternocleidomastoideus
Regio cervicalis lateralis	posterior edge of the M. sternocleidomastoideus, anterior edge of the M. trapezius, upper edge of the clavicula
Trigonum omotrapezoideum	posterior edge of the M. sternocleidomastoideus, anterior edge of the M. trapezius, upper edge of the M. omohyoideus (Venter inferior)
Trigonum omoclaviculare	posterior edge of the M. sternocleidomastoideus, upper edge of the clavicula, lower edge of the M. omohyoideus (Venter inferior)

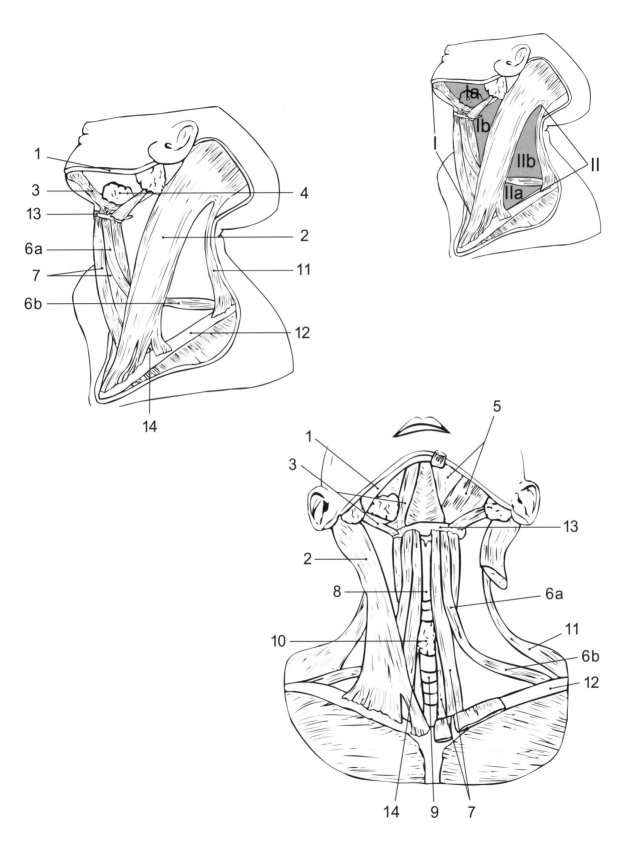

Abb. 8.1

8.2 Cervical Plexus

The **Rr. anteriores of the spinal nerves** form networks (so-called **plexus**) in the area of certain spinal cord segments. Here in the neural fibres of the Rr. anteriores connect to networks, so that the peripheral nerves which arise from the plexus contain neural fibres from several spinal cord segments. In the case of the **Plexus cervicalis**, the anterior branches of the spinal nerves **C1–C4/5** form the network from which the peripheral nerves of the Plexus cervicalis arise. Muscular and cutaneous branches of the Plexus cervicalis can be differentiated.

Muscular branches They provide short branches to the deep neck muscles (not shown) before the Rr. anteriores C1–C4/5 form the Plexus cervicalis.

The largest muscular branches of the Plexus cervicalis itself are the **Ansa cervicalis profunda** and the **N. phrenicus**. The **Ansa cervicalis profunda (1)** consists of a **Radix superior (1a)**, which is formed from the anterior branches of the spinal nerves C1/C2. The Radix superior runs transitionally along with the **N. hypoglossus (N. XII, 2)** and then unites with the **Radix inferior (1b)** from C2–3. The Ansa cervicalis profunda innervates the infrahyoidal muscles.

The **N. phrenicus (3)** contains neural fibres from C3–5. It runs along the neck, ascending into the thorax and innervates the diaphragm (phren) as well as other structures.

Cutaneous branches The so-called **Punctum nervosum (Erb's point, 5)** is situated on the posterior edge of the **M. sternocleidomastoideus (4)** in the Regio cervicalis lateralis (➤ Chap. 8.1). At this point, the cutaneous branches of the Plexus cervicalis reach the surface and fan out into different directions:

- **N. occipitalis minor**
- **N. auricularis magnus**
- **N. transversus colli**
- **Nn. supraclaviculares**

The **N. occipitalis minor (6)** contains neural fibres from C2. It ascends at the posterior edge of the M. sternocleidomastoideus and supplies the skin in the area of the lateral occiput.

The **N. auricularis magnus (7)** contains the neural fibres from C2–3. It runs obliquely via the M. sternocleidomastoideus cranially and innervates the skin in front of and behind the external ear.

The **N. transversus colli (8)** contains neural fibres from C2–3. It crosses over the M. sternocleidomastoideus in a medial direction and thereby reaches the skin of the anterior neck area.

Together with the **R. colli of the N. facialis (9)**, it there forms the **Ansa cervicalis superficialis (10)** , which innervates the **platysma (11)**.

The **Nn. supraclaviculares (12)** contain neural fibres from C3–4. They spread fanlike caudally to the skin over the clavicula, the shoulder and the chest.

The **N. accessorius (N. XI, 13)** also reaches the surface in the Regio cervicalis lateralis and runs dorsally to the M. trapezius. The N. accessorius is a cranial nerve and only has topographical proximity to the Plexus cervicalis.

> **Note**
>
> **Plexus** are exclusively formed by **anterior branches of the spinal nerves**, and in the case of the Plexus cervicalis, by the anterior branches of the spinal nerves C1–C4/5.
>
> In the area of **Erb's point,** the cutaneous branches of the Plexus cervicalis reach the surface. They are there closely situated to the 11th cranial nerve (N. accessorius).

> **Clinical remarks**
>
> The N. phrenicus innervates the most important respiratory muscle with the diaphragm. **Lesions of the N. phrenicus** or its roots (C3–5) can therefore lead to **significantly restricted breathing**, and, in the case of bilateral paralysis, to life-threatening respiratory distress. **Phrenic nerve paralysis** can for instance be caused by obstetric trauma (avulsion of the spinal nerve root), tumours or operations.

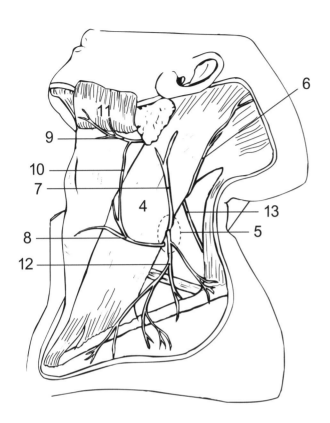

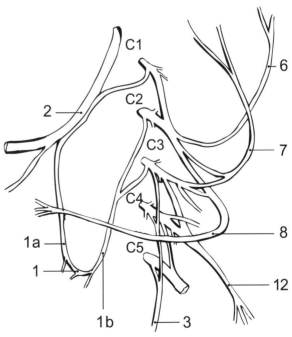

Abb. 8.2

8.3 Submandibular triangle

The Trigonum submandibulare is confined by the lower edge of the **mandibula (1)** as well as by the **Venter anterior (2a)** and the **Venter posterior (2b)** of the **M. digastricus**. The Venter posterior of the M. digastricus penetrates the parallel-running **M. stylohyoideus (3)**. Both the bellies of the M. digastricus are connected through an intermediate tendon, which is attached to the **Os hyoideum (4)**. In the depths of the Trigonum submandibulare lie the muscles of the floor of the mouth, of which the **M. mylohyoideus (5)** and the **M. hyoglossus (6)** are visible. In the superficial layer of the Trigonum submandibulare is the **Gl. submandibularis (7)**, a salivary gland, which empties under the tongue.

Nerve branches   Parallel to the lower edge of the mandibula, the **R. marginalis mandibulae (8)** leaves the N. facialis (N. VII). It innervates the mimetic muscles in this area. Slightly below (as early as in the Trigonum submandibulare) the **N. mylohyoideus (9)** runs in the direction of the chin. It innervates the eponymously named muscle and the Venter anterior of the M. digastricus. The N. mylohyoideus originates from the Portio minor of the N. mandibularis (N. V/3).

The **N. hypoglossus (N. XII, 10)** is situated in the neck, initially in the Trigonum caroticum, then turns cranially and runs below the tendons of the Venter posterior of the M. digastricus and the M. stylohyoideus into the Trigonum submandibulare. There it disappears just above the M. mylohyoideus, to reach the tongue which it supplies with motor innervation.

The **N. lingualis** runs cranially far into the depths, hidden by the Gl. submandibularis. It reaches into the triangle with just a short arch and turns around cranially and rostrally. Thus it travels above the floor of the mouth to the tongue, where it provided sensory innervation anterior two-thirds. Accompanying it is the **Chorda tympani** from the N. facialis (N. VII). It carries sensory fibres providing taste sensation to the anterior two-thirds of the tongue and the preganglionic parasympathetic fibres. These end in the Trigonum submandibulare at the eponymously-named **ganglion** and innervate, amongst others, the Gl. submandibularis.

Arteries and veins   Also in the Trigonum caroticum, the **A. lingualis (12)** originates from the **A. carotis externa (11).** It runs into the Trigonum submandibulare and eventually into the area of the floor of the mouth and the tongue. The **A. facialis (13)** is also a branch of the A. carotis externa, which runs through the Trigonum submandibulare. It reaches the triangle further cranially and dorsally than the A. lingualis and is most-

ly hidden there by the Gl. submandibularis. There the **A. submentalis (14)** also branches out of the A. facialis, which runs together with the N. mylohyoideus below the mandibula. The A. facialis crosses over the lower edge of the mandibula and thereby reaches the facial area. There it lies superficially and its pulse is palpable on the anterior edge of the M. masseter. Next to it is the **V. facialis (15)**. It does nevertheless run via the Gl. submandibularis and empties in the Trigonum caroticum into the **V. jugularis interna (16)**.

> **Note**
>
> The following important structures are in the Trigonum submandibulare:
> - **A./V. submentalis, A./V. facialis** and **A./V. lingualis**
> - **N. hypoglossus, N. mylohyoideus, N. lingualis, Chorda tympani** and **Ganglion submandibulare**
> - **Gl. submandibularis** as well as
> - **submandibular lymph nodes**

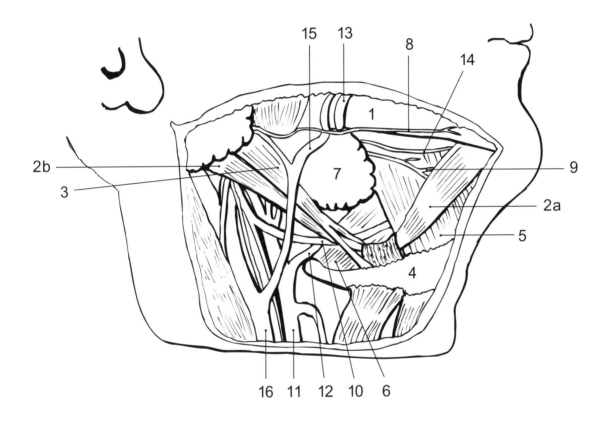

Abb. 8.3

163

8.4 Carotid triangle

The **Carotid triangle (Trigonum caroticum) (I)** is confined by the lower margin of the **Venter posterior of the M. digastricus (1)**, the upper margin of the **Venter superior of the M. omohyoideus (2)** and the anterior margin of the **M. sternocleidomastoideus (3)**. If the platysma as well as the superficial and middle cervical fascia are dissected and the M. sternocleidomastoideus is pulled slightly dorsally with a hook, the carotid sheath of the neck becomes visible in the Trigonum caroticum.

A. carotis communis   The **A. carotis communis (4)** runs in the carotid sheath of the neck. Its bifurcation in the **A. carotis externa (5)** and the **A. carotis interna (6)** lies in the Trigonum caroticum. While the A. carotis interna runs to the skull base without any further emission of branches, the A. carotis externa already provides its initial branches in the Trigonum caroticum:

- Firstly, the **A. thyroidea superior (7)** provides the **A. laryngea superior (8)** , which runs to the larynx. Subsequently the A. thyroidea superior runs ventral-medially to the thyroid gland.
- As the second branch of the A. carotis externa, the **A. lingualis (9)** runs cranial-ventrally in the direction of the Trigonum submandibulare (➤ Chap. 8.3) and the floor of the mouth.
- The **A. pharyngea ascendens**   (not visible), the small **R. sternocleidomastoideus** and the **A. facialis** also branch off in the Trigonum caroticum from the A. carotis externa.

V. jugularis interna   The **V. jugularis interna (10)** runs together with the A. carotis in the carotid sheath and incorporate various branches in the Trigonum caroticum, including the **V. facialis (11)**.

Nerves   The **N. vagus (N. X, 12)** runs along the carotid sheath between the A. carotis and the V. jugularis interna. In this area, it provides the N. laryngeus superior to the larynx (not shown) and then runs further downward to the upper thoracic aperture.

In the Trigonum caroticum, the **Ansa cervicalis profunda (13)** also emerges from the Plexus cervicalis with its **Radix inferior (13a)** and **Radix superior (13b)**. The **Radix superior** partially accompanies the 12th cranial nerve, the **N. hypoglossus (14)**. This nevertheless turns round in as early as the cranial part of the Trigonum caroticum, runs below the **M. stylohyoideus (15)** and the Venter posterior of the **M. digastricus (1)** and thereby reaches the Trigonum submandibulare.

Note

In the **Trigonum caroticum** are the following important structures:
- **A. carotis communis,** which branches off into the A. carotis interna and A. carotis externa as well as the initial outflows of the A. carotis externa
- **V. jugularis interna** with its tributaries
- **N. vagus, N. hypoglossus** and **Ansa cervicalis profunda**.

Clinical remarks

In the Trigonum caroticum it is possible to feel the **arterial pulse of the A. carotis communis (carotid pulse)**. This palpation point is particularly suited for assessing a weak arterial pulse.

The **Glomus caroticum,** a neural structure which registers the pH-value such as the oxygen and carbon dioxide content via **chemoreceptors** is located at the bifurcation of the A. carotis communis.

In the extended initial part of the A. carotis interna **(carotid sinus)** there are **baroreceptors** in walls of the blood vessels, which take part in the reflexive regulation of blood pressure. Patients with a **hypersensitive carotid sinus** need very little external manual stimulation in this area (e.g. with shaving, turning the head or feeling of the pulse) to trigger a reflexive lowering of blood pressure causing vertigo or syncope.

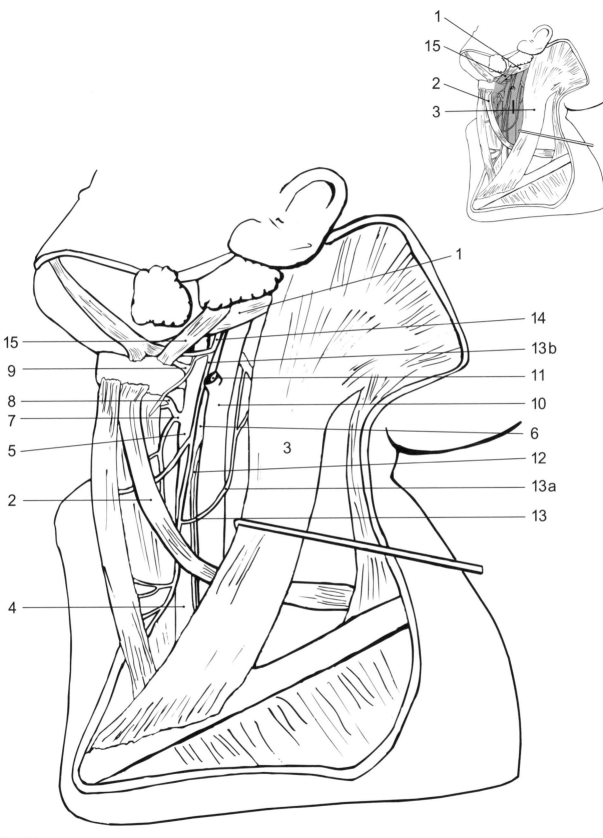

Abb. 8.4

8.5 Deep neck area

The **M. sternocleidomastoideus (1)** has been removed down to its origin to show the structures in the depths of the Trigonum caroticum and in the lateral neck area. The fascia of the neck and parts of the **V. jugularis interna (2)**, the **A. carotis communis (3)** as well as the **Aa. carotides interna (4)** and **externa (5)** were also removed.

Truncus sympathicus The **Truncus sympathicus (sympathetic trunk)** becomes visible. Behind the A. carotis, it shows thicker parts which correspond with paravertebral sympathetic ganglia (clusters of sympathetic neural cell bodies). In the neck area there are three ganglia of the sympathetic trunk: Ganglia cervicalia superius, medium and inferius.
The **Ganglion cervicale superius (6a)** lies at the level of the 2nd–4th cervical vertebrae (not shown). The **Ganglion cervicale medium (6b)** is in close topographical proximity to the **A. thyroidea inferior (7).** The lower cervical ganglion (not shown) often fuses with the upper thoracic ganglion to the **Ganglion stellatum** (➤ Chap. 8.6).
The cervical sympathetic trunk distributes small branches which are not shown here: from the top cervical ganglion, fine neural networks run along the branches of the Aa. carotides interna and externa to cranial and sympathetically innervate the soft tissue of the head as well as parts of the intraocular eye muscles. Shorter branches of the cervical sympathetic trunk run to the viscera of the neck and longer descending branches supply the thoracic organs.
The **N. vagus (N. X, 8)** also becomes more visible by removing the large cervical vessels. It runs, coming from the base of the skull, to the upper thoracic aperture. The N. vagus already provides in the area of the neck numerous small branches (not shown), which parasympathetically innervate the viscera of the neck and the thoracic organs.

Plexus cervicalis The **Ansa cervicalis profunda** already becomes partially visible (➤ Chap. 8.4) after a superficial dissection of the neck area. On this illustration, it is possible to see, in the depths next to the **Radix superior (9a),** the origin of the **Radix inferior (9b)** from the **Plexus cervicalis (10)**.
The **N. phrenicus (11)** also originates from the lower segments of the Plexus cervicalis and proceeds onto the **M. scalenus anterior (12)** to the upper thoracic aperture. It innervates, amongst others, the most important respiratory muscle, the diaphragm (phren), as well as sensory parts of the pleura, the peritoneum and the pericardium.

Further branches of the Plexus cervicalis which are visible, are the **N. occipitalis minor (13)** and the **Nn. supraclaviculares (14)**, severed here, which innervate the skin via the clavicula.

A. subclavia The **A. subclavia (15)** is visible in the area of the upper thoracic aperture. Where it bends, it provides the **A. thoracica interna (16)** and the **Truncus thyreocervicalis (17)** . The **A. thyroidea inferior (7)** arises here, supplying the Gl. thyroidea (thyroid gland) together with the **A. thyroidea superior (18)** from the A. carotis externa. Subsequently the **A. subclavia (15)** runs together with the **trunci of the Plexus brachialis (19)** through the scalene gap between the **Mm. scaleni anterior (12)** and **medius (20)** in the direction of the axilla.
The **N. accessorius (21)** can be seen in the lateral neck area. It descends from the base of the skull below the **M. trapezius (22)**.

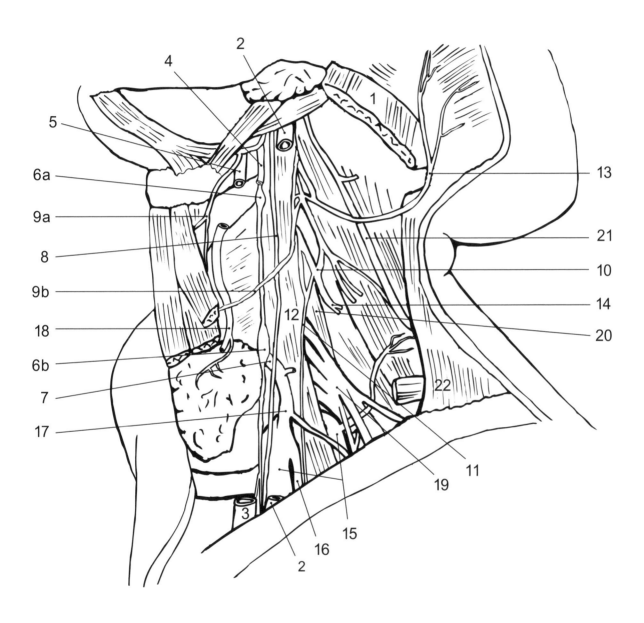

Abb. 8.5

8.6 Deep neck area and upper thoracic aperture

Deep cervical muscles The Spatium prevertebrale of the neck becomes visible after dissecting all structures from ventral up to and including the deep fascia of the neck. Here are the deep cervical muscles, of which the **M. longus colli (1)** as well as the **Mm. scaleni anterior (2)** and **medius (3)** are distinguishable in the illustration. The prevertebral muscles are involved with bending the head and the cervical spine to the front and to the side. The Mm. scaleni raises the ribs.

Truncus sympathicus The **Truncus sympathicus (sympathetic trunk, 4)** lies on the prevertebral muscles of the neck. It consists of clusters of sympathetic neural cell bodies (ganglia) as well as of their commissural neural fibres. The ganglia in the area of the neck are closely connected to the Rr. anteriores of the spinal nerves which form the Plexus brachialis and the Plexus cervicalis. Of the ganglia, the **Ganglion cervicale medium (5)** and the **Ganglion cervicale inferius** are visible. These often fuse with the top thoracic sympathetic trunk ganglion of the **Ganglion stellatum (6).** The Ganglion stellatum lies in the upper thoracic aperture in close proximity to the outflow of the **A. vertebralis (7)** from the **A. subclavia (8).** The A. vertebralis, which ascends into the Foramina transversalia of the thoracic vertebrae, only becomes visible after removal of the prevertebral muscles.

Plexus cervicalis and brachialis The Rr. anteriores of the spinal nerves, which form the **Plexus cervicalis (9),** are located in the Spatium prevertebrale. From here, amongst others, emerges the **N. phrenicus (10),** which descends in the upper thoracic aperture.
The **trunci and fasciculi of the Plexus brachialis (11)** run from the Spatium prevertebrale together with the **A. subclavia (8)** via the scalene gap behind the **M. scalenus anterior (2)** to the axilla.

Upper thoracic aperture On the lower half of the illustration, the course of the large arteries near the heart, coming from the upper thoracic aperture, can be seen. These continue in different directions: on the right side of the body, the **Truncus brachiocephalicus (13)** emerges from the **Arcus aortae (12);** on the left side of the body, the **A. carotis communis (14)** and the **A. subclavia (8)** branch off.

In the area of the upper thoracic aperture, the **pleura dome and the apex of the lung (15)** reach into the neck area and lie there in the Fossa supraclavicularis major.

Note

The following important structures lie in the deep neck area in and underneath the deep cervical fascia:
- the **prevertebral muscles**
- the **Truncus sympathicus**
- the **Rr. anteriores of the Nn. spinales,** which form the Plexus cervicalis and the Plexus brachialis

Clinical remarks

The pleural domes and the apices of the lungs reach into the Fossa supraclavicularis major at the neck. With the placement of a **central venous catheter** in the V. subclavia it should therefore be noted that accidental puncturing of the pleural dome can lead to air entering the pleural space and can cause a **collapsed lung (pneumothorax)**.
Because of their close proximity, **tumours of the apex of the lung** can infiltrate the structures of the deep neck area such as the trunci of the Plexus brachialis or the sympathetic trunk. In this way, lung tumours can cause **radiating pain in the arm** or **loss of sympathetic innervation to the head (Horner's syndrome)**.

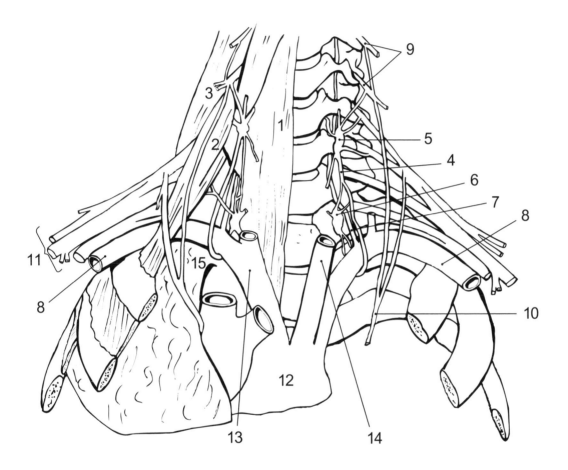

Abb. 8.6

8.7 Laryngeal skeleton and muscles

The five most important cartilages of the laryngeal skeleton are the large, unpaired

- **Cartilago thyroidea (thyroid cartilage)**
- **Cartilago cricoidea (cricoid cartilage)**
- **Cartilago epiglottica (epiglottis)**

as well as the small, paired

- **Cartilagines arytenoideae (arytenoid cartilage)**

Ventral view In this view, the **Cartilago thyroidea (thyroid cartilage, 1a–d)** can be seen. It consists of two **laminae (1a),** which are connected in the midline with each other and which form an angle. In the cranial part of this angle, the **Incisura thyroidea superior (1b)** cuts into the thyroid cartilage. In this area, the thyroid cartilage protrudes furthest ventrally and is palpable in men as the **Prominentia laryngea (Adam's apple)**.

By projecting over its upper edge, and with the lateral and upwards reaching **Cornua superiora (1c),** the thyroid cartilage is in contact with the **Corpus (2a)** and the **Cornua majora (2b)** of the **Os hyoideum (hyoid bone)**: the **Membrana thyrohyoidea (3)** spans the space between the thyroid cartilage and the hyoid bone. In it is the **Foramen n. laryngei superioris (4),** an opening for the R. internus of the N. laryngeus superior and the A. laryngea superior into the inner larynx.

The **Cartilago cricoidea (cricoid cartilage, 5a and b)** adjoin caudally of the thyroid cartilage. The narrower **arcus of the Cartilago cricoidea (5a)** can be seen from ventral, connected to the thyroid cartilage via the **Lig. cricothyroideum (6)**. Laterally, the capsule of the **Articulatio cricothyroidea (7)** is visible. In this articulated connection, the cricoid cartilage connects with the **Cornua inferiora (1d)** of the thyroid cartilage: the cricoid cartilage can be tilted against the thyroid cartilage in these joints. This movement is carried out by the **M. cricothyroideus,** of which the **Pars obliqua (8a)** and the **Pars recta (8b)** are visible. It is innervated as the only laryngeal muscle by the R. externus of the N. laryngeus superior. The cricoid cartilage is connected to the first **cartilage of the trachea (Cartilagines tracheales, 10)** via the **Lig. cricotracheale (9)**.

Dorsal view In this view, the thyroid cartilage (1a–d), the hyoid bone (2a–b) and the **lamina of the cricoid cartilage (5b),** which resembles the seal of a signet ring, can be seen.
In the middle, the **epiglottis (11)** projects into the inner larynx behind the hyoid bone, the Membrana thyrohyoidea and the thyroid cartilage. The epiglottis consists of elastic cartilage.

With a swallowing action it is pressed by the base of the tongue onto the laryngeal aperture and thereby closes the airways. Its lateral edges converge to dorsal and run along the **Cartilagines arytenoideae (arytenoid cartilage, 12)**. Thereby the Plica aryepiglottica, which is covered in mucosa, is raised in the larynx. The pyramidal arytenoid cartilage sits on the upper edge of the widened lamina of the cricoid cartilage. They have a Processus vocalis which faces ventrally and a Processus muscularis which faces laterally (not shown). The arytenoid cartilage is articulately connected with the cricoid cartilage and can in this way slide away from it and rotate on it. These movements are induced via the inner laryngeal muscles, which are innervated by the N. laryngeus inferior from the N. laryngeus recurrens. Of these, the **M. arytenoideus transversus (13),** which converges with the arytenoid cartilage, can be seen. The **M. arytenoideus obliquus (14)** also converges with the arytenoid cartilage and tilts it inwards on the cricoid cartilage. The **M. cricoarytenoideus posterior (15)** inserts from dorsal on the Proc. muscularis of the arytenoid cartilage and turns it outwards. Its antagonist is the M. cricoarytenoideus lateralis (not shown), which inserts from ventral on the Processus muscularis of the arytenoid cartilage and turns it inwards. From the arytenoid cartilages, the **M. aryepiglotticus (16)** runs to the epiglottis. It takes part in closing the glottis.

The contraction of the various laryngeal muscles does not only enable the opening or the closing of the glottis, and phonation or respiration. An altered tension of the vocal cords additionally induces a change in the pitch level with phonation. The only muscle that opens the glottis is the M. cricoarytenoideus posterior **(posterior cricoarytenoid muscle).**

Clinical remarks

The cartilaginous laryngeal skeleton can, particularly with older people, become partially ossified and then becomes visible in X-ray images of the neck.
With an obstruction of the airways or with the placing of a tracheal tube in long-term ventilation, the usual approach is to enter operatively between the tracheal cartilages **(tracheotomy)**. In emergency situations, opening the airways via the Ligamentum cricothyroideum **(coniotomy)** is advisable.

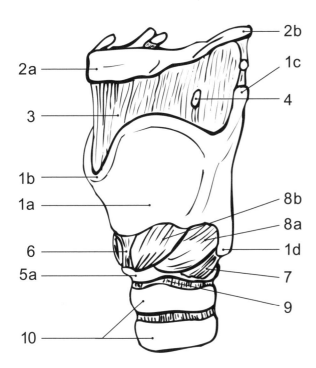

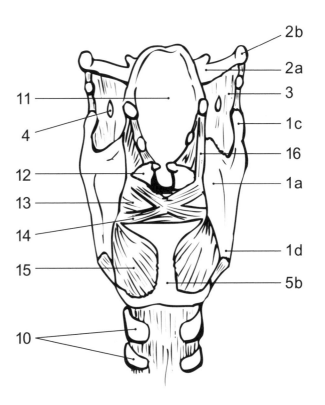

Abb. 8.7

8.8 Inner surface of the larynx

It is possible to see, when looking at the frontal and sagittal section, that the larynx is subdivided into three levels by two overlapping mucosal folds, the respectively paired **Plica vestibularis (vestibular fold, 1)** and **Plica vocalis (vocal fold, 2)**.

Upper level of the larynx   The **Vestibulum laryngis (I)** forms the upper level and connects with the laryngopharynx to dorsal. The entrance to the larynx (**Aditus laryngis**) is confined ventrally by the **epiglottis (3)**, laterally by the **Plicae aryepiglotticae (4)** and dorsally by the **Cartilagines arytenoideae (arytenoid cartilage, 5)**. Caudally the Vestibulum laryngis extends to the **Plicae vestibulares (1)**.

Middle level of the larynx   The middle level consists of the **Rima glottidis (glottis, 6)** which lies between the Plicae vocales (2), and both of the lateral mucosal recesses between the Plica vestibularis and the Plica vocalis (**Ventriculi laryngis, 7**). Both of the **Plicae vocales (2)** form the **glottis (II)**. The elastic **Ligamenta vocalia (vocal cords, 8)** and the striated **Mm. vocales (9)** lie in the Plicae vocales.

Lower level of the larynx   Below the Plicae vocales is the lower level of the larynx (**Cavum infraglotticum, III**), which is connected caudally with the trachea.

Larynx muscles and support system   The muscles of the larynx are somatomotor in innervation and striated. Besides the **Mm. vocales (9),** the other laryngeal muscles that can be seen are the **Mm. cricothyroideus (10)**, the **Mm. cricoarythenoidei laterales (11)** and the **Mm. aryepiglottici (12)**. With the exception of the M. cricothyroideus, which is innervated by the N. laryngeus superior, all other laryngeal muscles are supplied by the N. laryngeus recurrens. The mucous membrane of the larynx is innervated above the Plicae vocales by the N. laryngeus superior, and below by the N. laryngeus inferior. In the frontal and sagittal section, the **Os hyoideum (13)**, the **Cartilago thyroidea (14)** and the **Cartilago cricoidea (15)** are visible.

Phonation   The inner muscles of the larynx can close the Rima glottidis completely. This is important for phonation: while the Rima glottidis is opened with respiration, breathing out takes place with a **closed glottis** during phonation. This leads to horizontal oscillations of the vocal cords, thereby forming tones. The **contraction of the Mm. vocales** leads to a change in the tension of the vocal cords and thereby induces a change in pitch.

Clinical remarks

The mucous membrane of the larynx sits on loose connective tissue in the area of the Plicae vestibulares. This favours the forming of an oedema (sharp increase of interstitial fluid) in the case of **insect bites** in this area or in the context of a **general allergic reaction**. Oedema can progress to such a degree that the airways are completely obstructed, necessitating an emergency airway puncture below the glottis **(coniotomy)**.

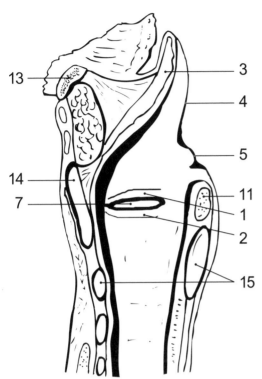

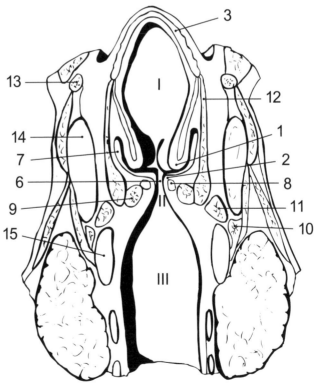

Abb. 8.8

8.9 Upper airways and digestive tract

On the median sagittal section through the head and the neck, the upper airways can be seen:

- **Cavitas nasi (nasal cavity, I)**
- **Pharynx (pharynx, IIa–c)**
- **Larynx (IIIa–c)**
- **upper trachea (wind-pipe, IV)**

It is also possible to see the beginning of the digestive tract:

- **Cavitas oris (oral cavity, V)**
- **Pharynx (IIa–c)**
- **cranial oesophagus (VI)**

Cavitas nasi (I)   The nasal cavity has been opened and the **Septum nasi (1),** which is covered with mucosa, is visible. In the anterior area it is cartilaginous and in the posterior part it is bony. The nasal cavity is separated from the oral cavity by the **hard palate (2)** and the **soft palate (3).** To dorsal, the nasal cavity is in contact with the upper level of the pharynx, the **nasopharynx (IIa),** via the choanae.

Cavitas oris (V)   The oral cavity can be subdivided into the oral vestibule (Vestibulum oris) and the actual oral cavity (Cavitas oris propria): the **Vestibulum oris (4)** lies between the cheeks and/or the lips and the dental arches. The **Cavitas oris propria** lies inside the dental arches and is filled largely by the **tongue (5).** To dorsal, the oral cavity is in contact with the middle level of the pharynx, the **oropharynx (IIb),** via the narrow **Isthmus faucium (VII),** which is formed by the palatal arches.

Pharynx (IIa–c)   The pharynx belongs to the airways as well as to the digestive tract. It consists of three levels, the **nasopharynx (epipharynx, IIa),** the **oropharynx (mesopharynx, IIb)** and the **laryngopharynx (hypopharynx, IIc).**
The walls of the pharynx are formed by the pharyngeal muscles. The interior space of the pharynx is covered with mucosa. The **Ostium pharyngeum tubae auditivae (6),** the opening of the Tuba auditiva which ventilates the tympanic cavity, is located in the nasopharynx. Directly next to this opening is the **Tonsilla pharyngealis (pharyngeal tonsil, 7)** which consists of lymphatic tissue.
The oropharynx is in contact with the oral cavity. Lymphatic tissue, the **Tonsilla palatina (palatal tonsil, 8)** also lies between both arches which border the **Isthmus faucium (VII).**
The **laryngopharynx (IIc)** forms the bottom level of the pharynx and lies directly dorsal of the laryngeal aperture. It continues caudally into the cervical part of the **oesophagus (VI).** In

the area of the laryngopharynx, the upper airway and the digestive tract intersect each other.

Larynx (IIIa–c)   The laryngeal aperture (Aditus laryngis) is in front of the laryngopharynx and allows access to the **Vestibulum laryngis (IIIa).** The **Ventriculus laryngis (IIIb)** bulges out on both sides in the area of the glottis, between the **Plica vestibularis (9)** and the **Plica vocalis (10)** . Below the Plica vocalis, the **infraglottic space (IIIc)** continues without interruption into the **trachea (IV).**

Act of swallowing   As the upper airways and digestive tract communicate with each other and intersect in the area of the laryngopharynx, it is essential that no food ends up in the nasal cavity and/or in the larynx and trachea when swallowing. Initially when swallowing, the tongue pushes the food in the direction of the oropharynx. Simultaneously, the contraction of the upper pharyngeal muscles and the muscles of the soft palate induce the closing of the oropharynx to the nasopharynx. The dorsal movement of the tongue and the upward movement of the larynx lead to the **epiglottis (11)** being pressed down by the **base of the tongue (5a)** onto the Aditus laryngis. Thereby the epiglottis folds over the Vestibulum laryngis and closes the airways. Food can now be transported past the epiglottis into the digestive tract, which takes over the reflex contraction of the middle and lower pharyngeal muscles.

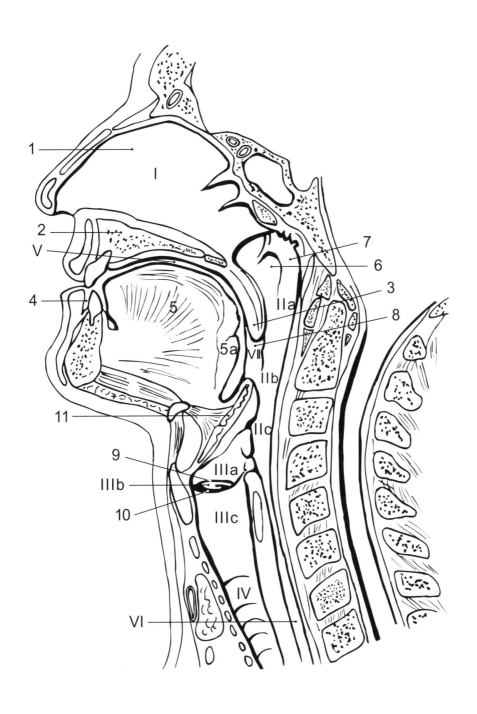

Abb. 8.9

175

9.1 Brain, lateral view

The cerebrum is subdivided into a right and a left hemisphere. Each hemisphere is divided into the following lobes:

- **Lobus frontalis (frontal lobe, A)**
- **Lobus temporalis (temporal lobe, B)**
- **Lobus parietalis (parietal lobe, C)**
- **Lobus occipitalis (occipital lobe, D)**

The cerebral hemisphere has a convex shape on the lateral surface and crosses over on the **side of the mantle (1)** into the straight medial side. The **Lobus frontalis (A)**, the **Lobus temporalis (B)**, the **Lobus parietalis (C)** and the **Lobus occipitalis (D)** can be seen on the convex surface. The surface of the cerebrum is greatly increased by the presence of **gyri** and **sulci**. Although there are interindividual variants, there are general rules for the location of the gyri and sulci.

Lobus frontalis   The **Lobus frontalis (frontal lobe, A)** lies rostrally of the **Sulcus centralis (2)** and above the deep **Sulcus lateralis (3)**. On the Lobus frontalis, two sulci run in a sagittal direction, the **Sulci frontales superior (4)** and **inferior (5)**.
The sulci frontales separate three gyri which extend in rostro-caudal direction from the **frontal pole (6)** to the **Sulcus lateralis (2)**: the **Gyri frontales superior (A1)**, **medius (A2)** und **inferior (A3)**. The Gyrus frontalis inferior is subdivided by the **Rr. anterior (3a)** and **ascendens (3b)** of the Sulcus lateralis into a **Pars orbitalis (A3.1)**, **Pars triangularis (A3.2)** and **Pars opercularis (A3.3)**. The Gyri frontales superior, medius and inferior are separated by the **Sulcus precentralis (7)** from the **Gyrus precentralis (A4),** lying directly rostral of the Sulcus centralis.

Lobus temporalis   The **Lobus temporalis (temporal lobe, B)** is separated from the Lobus frontalis by the **Sulcus lateralis (3)**. Two horizontal sulci, the **Sulci temporales superior (8)** and **inferior (9)**, run along the temporal lobe.
They border the **Gyri temporales superior (B1)**, **medius (B2)** and **inferior (B3)**. On the upper side of the Gyrus temporalis superior, the **Gyri temporales transversi** (not shown) run into the depths of the Sulcus lateralis.

Lobus parietalis   The **Lobus parietalis (parietal lobe, C)** lies behind the **Sulcus centralis (2)**. It continues occipitally in the Lobus occipitalis without sharp borders and is separated from the Lobus temporalis by the **Sulcus lateralis (3)**.
Behind the Sulcus centralis lies the **Gyrus postcentralis (C1)**, with which the **Sulcus postcentralis (10)** adjoins. It separates

the **Gyri parietales superior (C2)** and **inferior (C3)**, which are separated from each other by the **Sulcus intraparietalis (11)**. The **Gyrus supramarginalis (C4)** wraps around the occipital end of the Sulcus lateralis. The **Gyrus angularis (C5)** wraps around the end of the Sulcus temporalis superior.

Lobus occipitalis   Across the convexity of the cerebral hemisphere, the **Lobus occipitalis (occipital lobe, D)** passes without clear borders into the Lobus temporalis and the Lobus parietalis. The **Sulcus parietooccipitalis (12),** penetrating on the side of the **mantle (1)** and the **Incisura preoccipitalis (13)**, indicate the borders of the Lobus occipitalis.

> **Note**
>
> Certain cerebral cortex areas have allocated functions. In this way, the Gyrus precentralis represents the **primary motor cortex,** where the pyramidal tract commences.
> The ascending somatosensory tracts end in the **primary somatosensory cortex,** the Gyrus postcentralis.
> The **primary auditory cortex** is located in the Gyri temporales transversi (Heschl's gyri), in which the auditory pathway ends.

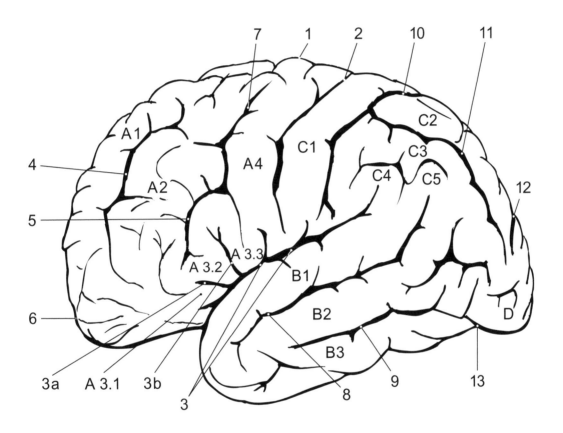

Abb. 9.1

177

9.2 Brain, medial view

After cutting both of the cerebral hemispheres with a median sagittal section, the telencephalon is visible on the medial side (the diencephalon and the brainstem have been removed here). This view shows the position of the commissures on one side and the gyri and the sulci of the cerebrum on the other side.

Commissures   Commissural fibres connect the two cerebral hemispheres with each other. The **Corpus callosum (1a–d)** is the biggest commissure. It starts with the **rostrum (1a)**, turns around occipitally in the **genu (knee, 1b)**, then continues in the **truncus (trunk, 1c)** and ends with the **splenium (1d)**.

A second, smaller commissure, the **Commissura anterior (2)**, adjoins at the **Rostrum corporis callosi (1a).**

Below the Corpus callosum a thin, transparent septum, the **Septum pellucidum (3)**, spreads itself out.

Medial surface of the cerebrum   On the **side of the mantle (4),** the convex, lateral surface passes over into the straight medial side. On this side, the **Sulcus centralis (5)** can be seen cutting into the side of the mantle. The **Gyrus paracentralis (6)** lies here along the Sulcus centralis. The **Sulci pre- (7)** and **postcentralis (8)** can be seen rostrally and/or occipitally of the Gyrus paracentralis, and in front of the Sulcus precentralis, the medial side of the **Gyrus frontalis superior (9)**. Parallel to the Corpus callosum, the **Sulcus cinguli (10)** runs below the Gyrus frontalis superior. Together with the Corpus callosum, it confines the **Gyrus cinguli (11)**.

The border between the Lobi parietalis and occipitalis can be seen on the medial surface. It is formed by the **Sulcus parietooccipitalis (12)**. Rostral of the Sulcus parietooccipitalis lies the **Precuneus (13)**, and occipitally thereof the wedge-shaped **cuneus (14)**. Below the cuneus runs a deeply penetrating sulcus into the Lobus occipitalis, the **Sulcus calcarinus (15)**.

The **Sulcus occipitotemporalis (16)** and the **Sulcus collateralis (17)** run lengthways on the bottom of the Lobi occipitalis and temporalis. From the outside inwards they border the **Gyri temporalis inferior (18), occipitotemporalis lateralis (19), occipitotemporalis medialis (20)** and **parahippocampalis (21).** The latter ends rostrally in the **uncus (22)**.

Note

Around the Sulcus calcarinus lies the primary visual cortex, where the visual pathway ends. A **retinotopic structure** is found in the primary visual cortex, i.e., certain cortex areas represent certain parts of the retina.

There is a similar **somatotopic structure** in the Gyri pre- and postcentralis, in which certain cortex areas are allocated to certain areas of the body.

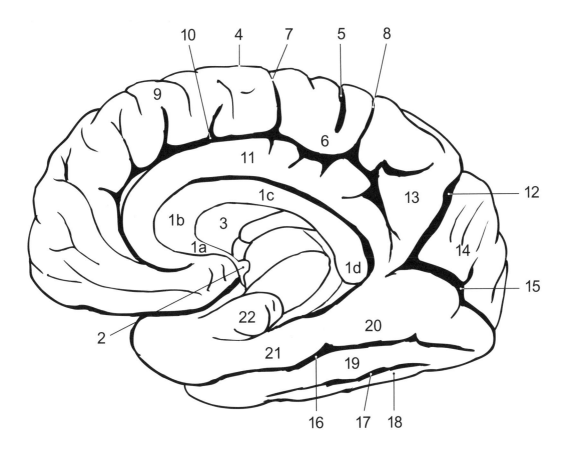

Abb. 9.2

179

9.3 Brain, basal view

In this view, the **cerebellum (A)**, the **brainstem (Truncus encephali, B1 und 2)**, parts of the **diencephalon (C1–3)** and the basal gyri and sulci of the cerebrum can be seen.

Cerebellum The **cerebellum (A)** lies below the Lobus occipitalis of the cerebrum and dorsally of the **brainstem (B)**. It is connected to the brainstem on each side respectively by three **cerebellar peduncles** (Pedunculi cerebelli, not shown). The cerebellar surface is more finely grooved than the cerebrum. Narrow gyri (**Folia cerebelli**) are visible, separated from each other with almost parallel running **Fissurae cerebelli**.

Brainstem The **brainstem (Truncus encephali, B1 and 2)** is subdivided into three parts:
- **mesencephalon (middle brain)**
- **pons (B1)**
- **myelencephalon (Medulla oblongata, afterbrain, B2)**

With regards to the **brainstem,** it is possible to see the **pons (B1),** which belongs to the metencephalon and the caudally adjoining **myelencephalon (B2)**. The brainstem is the exit point of the cranial nerves III–XII from the brain.
Furthest cranially, the **N. oculomotorius (N. III, 1)** emerges from the Fossa interpeduncularis of the mesencephalon (not shown).
As the only cranial nerve, the **N. trochlearis (N. IV, 2)** arises from the dorsal side of the brainstem, runs from there to ventral and becomes visible on the edge of the **pons (B1).**
The **N. trigeminus (N. V, 3a–d)** leaves the brain at the lateral border of the pons. A sensory ganglion, the **Ganglion trigeminale (3a)** can be seen, as well as the three branches of the N. trigeminus:
- **N. ophthalmicus (N. V/1, 3b)**
- **N. maxillaris (N. V/2, 3c)**
- **N. mandibularis (N. V/3, 3d)**

On the lower border of the pons, the **N. abducens (N. VI, 4)** is visible.
The **N. facialis (N. VII, 5)** and the **N. intermedius (5a)**, together with the **N. vestibulocochlearis (N. VIII, 6),** exit through the cerebellopontine angle.
Caudally of this group, the **N. glossopharyngeus (N. IX, 7)** and the **N. vagus (N. X, 8)** can be seen behind the olive.
Below the Nn. glossopharyngeus and vagus, the cranial roots of the **N. accessorius (N. XI, 9)** leave the Medulla oblongata and join the spinal roots of these nerves.

The **N. hypoglossus (N. XII, 10)** appears in front of the olive.

Diencephalon The **diencephalon (C1–3)** is mostly hidden by the cerebral hemispheres around the midline. In the basal view, the **Nn. optici (N. II, C1),** which belong to the diencephalon and join the **Chiasma opticum (C2),** are visible. Directly below the Chiasma opticum is the **pituitary (11)**. The **Corpora mammillaria (C3)** can be seen as a further structure of the diencephalon behind the pituitary.

Basal gyri of the cerebrum In the midline, the **Fissura longitudinalis cerebri (12)** can be seen, separating the two cerebral hemispheres from each other. On the basal surface of the Lobus frontalis runs the **Sulcus olfactorius (13),** which abuts the **N. olfactorius (N. I, 14).** Medial of the Sulcus olfactorius lies the **Gyrus rectus (15),** laterally the **Gyri** and **Sulci orbitales (16)**.

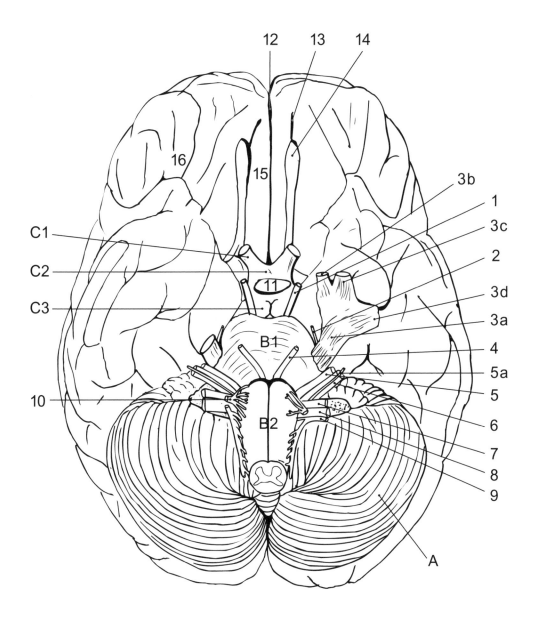

12 13 14

3b
1
3c
2
3d
3a
4
5a
5
6
7
8
9

C1
C2
C3

10

16
15

11

B1

B2

A

Abb. 9.3

181

9.4 Cerebellum and brainstem

After removal of the telencephalon and the diencephalon at the Pedunculi cerebri (cerebral peduncles), what is left is the lower brainstem with the mesencephalon and rhombencephalon (clinically speaking, the brainstem; the anatomic brainstem also encompasses the basal ganglia, ➤ Chap. 9.10 to ➤ Chap. 9.12). To dorsal, the brainstem (Truncus encephali) is connected via the cerebellar peduncles (Pedunculi cerebelli) with the **cerebellum (A).** With regards to the cerebellum, the **cerebellar hemispheres (A1)** are visible here, and laterally of the pons, the **flocculus (A2).**

Mesencephalon The **mesencephalon (middle brain, B1–6)** is the furthest cranial and shortest part of the brainstem. It connects the pons and the cerebellum with the cerebrum. On the basal side, the **Crus cerebri (B1)** can be seen, through which run numerous ascending and descending projection tracts. Between the two Crura cerebri is the **Fossa interpeduncularis (B2).** To dorsal, the Crura cerebri joins the **tegmentum (B3).**

The Crura cerebri and the tegmentum together form the **Pedunculi cerebri (cerebral peduncles, B4).** Dorsally of the tegmentum it is possible to see the narrow ventricular space of the mesencephalons, the **Aqueductus mesencephali (B5).** It connects the 3rd ventricle in the diencephalon with the 4th ventricle of the rhombencephalon (➤ Chap. 9.13). Dorsally of the aqueductus, the **tectum of the mesencephalon (B6)** adjoins.

The bottom illustration shows the view of a section through the **mesencephalon.** It is possible to recognise the structure in the **tectum (B6)** and the **tegmentum (B3)** – see the top illustration – and the **Aqueductus mesencephali (B5)** which lies in between. Basally, the **Crus cerebri (B1)** is visible, in which, amongst others, the Tractus corticospinalis (pyramidal tract) runs as an important, descending motor tract.

Dorsally, the **Substantia nigra (B7)** adjoins, connects functionally with the basal ganglia and possesses motor functions. Further dorsally is the **Nucleus ruber (B8),** which has a reddish color because of its high iron content and belongs to the extrapyramidal motor system. Directly ventral of the Aquaeductus mesencephali, there is a small section on the **Nucleus nervi oculomotorii** (IIIrd cranial nerve). Its exit from the brainstem is recognisable in the **Fossa interpeduncularis (B2).** Further along its course, it provides motor innervation to four of the outer eye muscles.

Dorsally of the aquaeductus is the **tectum (B6)** with the **quadrigeminal bodies.** Both of the truncated **Colliculi superiores (B9)** contain nuclear areas, responsible for reflex movements of the eyes and pupillary light reflexes. The **Colliculi inferiores** which lie underneath are not visible. They contain nuclear areas of the auditory pathway.

Parkinson's disease causes degeneration of dopaminergic neurons of the Substantia nigra. With the loss of a large part of these nerve cells, motoric disturbances develop such as a hypertonic **hypokinesis,** i.e. heightened muscle tone **(rigor)** accompanied by diminished movement (e.g. Parkinson's mask, small steps, decreased armswing, etc.). A further symptom of Parkinson's is the **resting tremor**.

Rhombencephalon The **rhombencephalon (hindbrain)** consists of two parts:
- cranial part: **metencephalon** with **cerebellum (A)** and **pons (C)**
- caudal part: **myelencephalon (D1–3)**

The pons is laterally in contact with the cerebellum via both of the **middle cerebellar peduncles (Pedunculi cerebellares medii, 1)** and is separated by the **Sulcus bulbopontinus (2)** from the myelencephalon.

On the ventral side of the myelencephalon, the **Fissura mediana anterior (D1)** and the **pyramids (Pyramides medullae oblongatae, D2)** can be seen. In the area of the **pyramidal decussation (Decussatio pyramidum, D2a),** fibres of the pyramidal tract cross to the opposite side. Laterally of the pyramids, the **olives (D3)** adjoin.

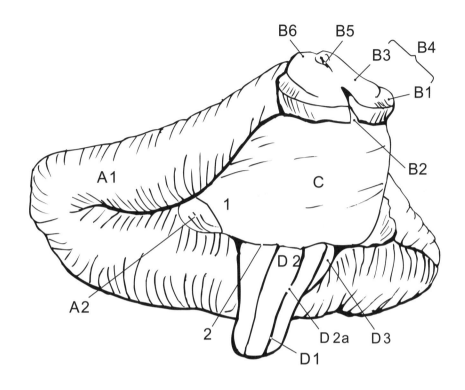

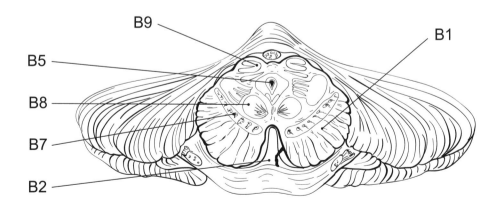

Abb. 9.4

183

9.5 Cranial nerve nuclei

Both these illustrations show the schematic position of the cranial nerve nuclei in the view from dorsal and lateral. The nuclei of the **cranial nerves III-XII** are in the **brainstem.** One differentiates:

- **Nuclei origines** containing neurons, which send out efferent neural fibres.
- Afferent, sensory tracts end in the **Nuclei terminationes**.

As is particularly clear in the dorsal view, the cranial nerve nuclei are systematically arranged.

Nuclei origines   In the dorsal view on the left side of the illustration:

- The **general somatoefferent nuclei** lie near the midline. They include the:
  - **Nuclei nervi oculomotorii (1;** N. III, in the mesencephalon, for the innervation of four of the outer eye muscles)
  - **Nuclei nervi trochlearis (2;** N. IV, in the mesencephalon, M. obliquus superior)
  - **Nuclei nervi abducentis (3;** N. VI, metencephalon, M. rectus lateralis)
  - **Nuclei nervi hypoglossi (4;** N. XII, myelencephalon, tongue muscles)
- The general visceroefferent (parasympathetic) nuclei lie slightly further laterally:
  - **Nuclei accessorius nervi oculomotorii (5;** N. III, mesencephalon, Mm. sphincter pupillae and ciliaris)
  - **Nuclei salivatorius superior (6;** N. VII, metencephalon, salivary glands on the floor of the mouth, lacrimal gland)
  - **Nuclei salivatorius inferior (7;** N. IX, myelencephalon, parotid gland)
  - **Nuclei dorsalis nervi vagi (8;** N. X, myelencephalon, viscera)
- Further laterally, the **specific visceroefferent nuclei** adjoin:
  - **Nuclei motorius nervi trigemini (9;** N. V, metencephalon, masticatory muscles)
  - **Nuclei nervi facialis (10;** N. VII, metencephalon, mimetic muscles)
  - **Nuclei ambiguus (11;** N. IX + X; myelencephalon, pharyngeal and laryngeal muscles)
  - **Nuclei nervi accessorii (12;** N. IX; myelencephalon/Medulla spinalis, Mm. trapezius and sternocleidomastoideus)

Nuclei terminationes   The laterally situated sensory **Nuclei terminationes** are subdivided into:

- General and specific visceroafferent nuclei
  - **Nuclei tractus solitarii (13)** with the **Pars inferior (13a;** N. IX + X, myeelencephalon, viscera) and the **Pars superior (13b;** N. VII + IX, myelencephalon, sense of taste)
- General somatoafferent nuclei
  - **Nuclei mesencephalicus nervi trigemini (14;** N. V, mesencephalon, proprioception of the masticatory muscles)
  - **Nuclei pontinus nervi trigemini (15;** N. V, metencephalon, epicritic sensitivity of the head)
  - **Nuclei spinalis nervi trigemini (16;** N. V + X, from the metencephalon up to the Medulla spinalis, protopathic sensitivity of the head)
- Specific somatoafferent nuclei
  - **Nuclei vestibulares superior (17a), lateralis (17b), medialis (17c)** and **inferior (17d).** All N. VIII, rhombencephalon, sense of balance.
  - **Nuclei cochleares anterior (18a)** and **posterior (18b).** Both N. VIII, metencephalon, hearing.

In the lateral view, besides the cranial nerve nuclei, the course of the neural fibres from and/or to their exit points from the brainstem can also be seen.

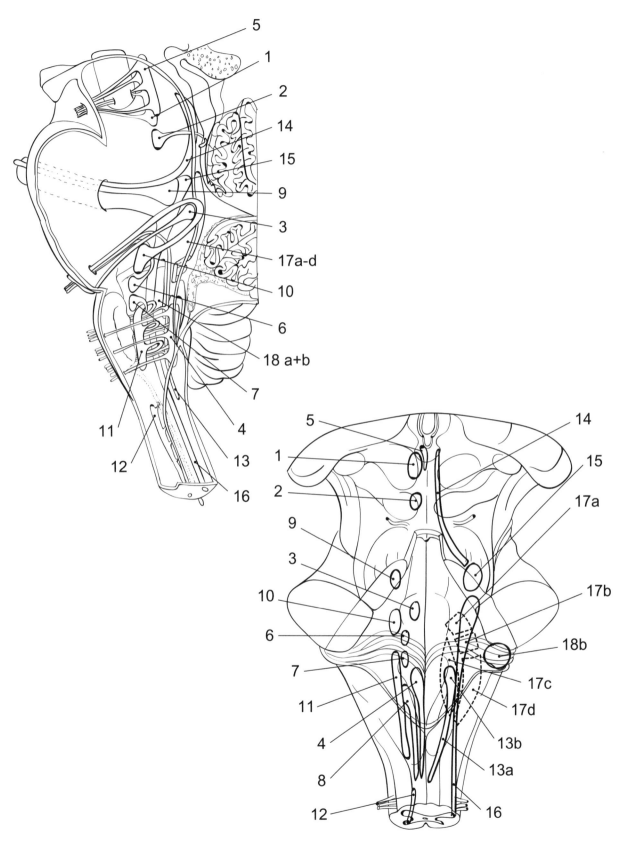

Abb. 9.5

9.6 Arteries of the brain, basal view

The arterial supply of the brain come from two sources:
- the two **Aa. vertebrales (1)** from the Aa. subclaviae
- the two **Aa. carotides internae (2)** from the Aa. carotides communes

The arteries are closed with the Aa. communicantes to form a **cerebral arterial circle (Circulus arteriosus cerebri)**.

Drainage area of the A. vertebralis The **A. vertebralis (1)** is the first branch of the A. subclavia. It ascends through the Foramina transversaria of the cervical vertebrae (➤ Chap. 7.10) and enters the skull via the Foramen magnum. When entering the base of the skull, the A. vertebralis lies ventrolaterally of the myelencephalon on the clivus. It provides the **A. inferior posterior cerebelli (3)** to the cerebellum and the **A. spinalis anterior (4)** to the myelencephalon and to the Medulla spinalis. Both of the Aa. spinales anteriores unite primarily into a trunk which descends in the Fissura mediana anterior.

On the border of the myelencephalon to the pons, both the Aa. vertebrales unite to become the **A. basilaris (5)**. This provides the **Aa. inferiores anteriores cerebelli (6)** and ascends itself in the midline to the upper border of the pons, where it supplies the pons with numerous short branches.

At the upper border of the pons, it provides the **Aa. superiores cerebelli (7)** in the Cisterna interpeduncularis to the upper side of the cerebellum and bifurcates immediately thereafter into its terminal branches, the **Aa. cerebri posteriores (8)**. These run around the Pedunculi cerebri and supply, amongst others, the Lobi occipitales and parts of the basal gyri of the Lobi temporales.

Drainage area of the A. carotis interna The **A. carotis interna (2)** is formed when the A. carotis communis divides at the neck (➤ Chap. 7.10). It runs without branching to the base of the skull and passes through the Canalis caroticus intracranially. Here it arrives at the basal surface of the brain, directly adjacent to the **pituitary gland (9)** and to the Sinus cavernosus (➤ Chap. 9.8). In this area, the A. carotis interna makes an S-shaped curve, the **carotid siphon**.

Directly after passing through the dura, the A. carotis interna provides the **A. ophthalmica** to the orbit (not shown). After providing numerous smaller branches, the A. carotis interna bifurcates into a medial terminal branch, the **A. cerebri anterior (10)**, and a lateral terminal branch, the **A. cerebri media (11)**.

The **A. cerebri anterior (10)** runs into the **Fissura longitudinalis cerebri (12)** and then in an arch on the Corpus callosum along the medial side of the cerebral hemisphere (➤ Chap. 9.7). Both of the Aa. cerebri anteriores are connected to each other before their entry into the Fissura longitudinalis cerebri via the **A. communicans anterior (13)**. In this way, the drainage areas of both of the Aa. carotides internae are connected to each other.

The **A. cerebri media (11)** runs laterally in front of the **insula (14)** into the depths of the Sulcus lateralis. Here it provides numerous branches, which amongst others also supply the basal ganglia and the Capsula interna (➤ Chap. 9.10 to ➤ Chap. 9.12). In the depths of the Sulcus lateralis, the A. cerebri media divides into a **Truncus superior (15)**, which supplies the convexity of the Lobi frontalis and parietalis, and a **Truncus inferior (16)**, which amongst others supplies the upper side and convexity of the Lobus temporalis.

Circulus arteriosus cerebri (Willisii) At the base of the brain, the drainage areas of both of the Aa. carotides internae are connected to each other and via the **A. communicans anterior (13)** as well as via the **A. communicans posterior (17)** with the A. basilaris. Thereby a cerebral arterial ring, the Circulus arteriosus cerebri (Circle of Willis), is formed. It presents strong interindividual varieties and appears in the shape depicted here only in approx. two-thirds of cases.

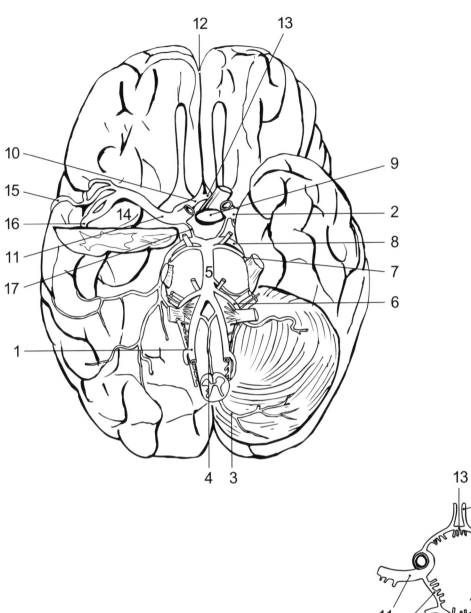

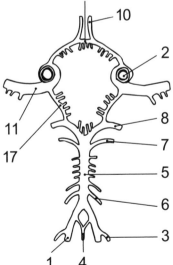

Abb. 9.6

187

9.7 Arteries of the brain, view from medial

The view from medial shows the areas supplied by the:
- **A. carotis interna (1)**
- **A. basilaris (2)**

A. carotis interna The **A. carotis interna (1)** can be seen below the **Chiasma opticum (3)**. The lateral terminal branch, the A. cerebri media, is hidden in the illustration. The medial terminal branch, the **A. cerebri anterior (4)**, turns rostrally in the Fissura longitudinalis cerebri. The A. cerebri anterior runs along the medial side of the cerebrum, ascending to the **Genu corporis callosi (5)** and runs from there occipitally in an arch adjacent to the Corpus callosum. With its branches, it supplies the medial side of the Lobi frontalis and parietalis. Its supply area extends over the **side of the mantle (6)** across the convexity of the cerebral hemisphere and ends occipitally in the area of the **precuneus (7)**.

A. basilaris The **A. basilaris (2)** is formed on the lower border of the **pons (8)** with the confluence of both of the **Aa. vertebrales (9)**. In the area of confluence, the **A. inferior posterior cerebelli (10)** flows out to the **cerebellum (11)**. The pons is supplied by numerous Rami ad pontes from the A. basilaris. At the level of the **Pedunculi cerebri (cerebral peduncles, 12)**, the A. basilaris is connected to the **A. communicans posterior (13)** with the drainage area of the A. carotis interna (Circulus arteriosus cerebri). Here the terminal branch of the A. basilaris, the **A. cerebri posterior (14)**, also turns round to dorsolateral and runs along the bottom of the Lobi temporalis and occipitalis. With its branches, it supplies the Lobus occipitalis and broad parts of the bottom of the temporal lobe.

Note

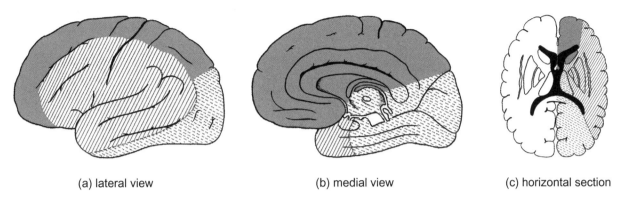

(a) lateral view   (b) medial view   (c) horizontal section

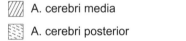

■ A. cerebri anterior

▨ A. cerebri media

▩ A. cerebri posterior

[aus Trepel, M. Neuroanatomie. Urban & Fischer, 3. Aufl., 2003]

Abb. 9.7   Supply areas of the large cranial arteries

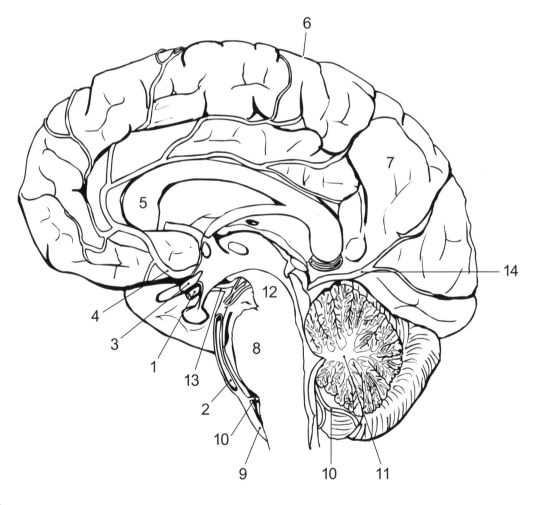

Abb. 9.8

9.8 Veins of the brain

The cranial veins can be divided into two groups:

- **Vv. cerebri superficiales** (outer cranial veins, superficial cranial veins), which drain the surface of the brain
- **Vv. cerebri profundae** (inner cranial veins, deep cranial veins), which drain the blood from deep cranial areas

The cranial veins do not have valves. Both venous systems are connected to each other by numerous anastomoses and eventually flow into the venous sinus of the dura mater (**Sinus durae matris**). The Sinus durae matris are valveless venous sinuses. They can be divided into:

- a dorsal group
- a ventral group

Dorsal group of the Sinus durae matris

To this group belongs the:

- **Sinus sagittalis superior (1)**
- **Confluens sinuum (2)**
- **Sinus sagittalis inferior (3)**
- **Sinus rectus (4)**
- **Sinus transversus (5)**
- **Sinus sigmoideus (6)**
- **Sinus occipitalis (7)**
- **Sinus marginalis** (not shown)

The **Sinus sagittalis superior (1)** begins frontally in the area of the Foramen caecum and runs along the midline in the area where the Falx cerebri attaches occipitally. It ends at the Protuberantia occipitalis interna in the **Confluens sinuum (2)**. Along its course, it incorporates numerous superficial cranial nerves, such as the **Vv. frontales (8)** and **parietales (9)**.

The **Sinus sagittalis inferior (3)** is contained in the inferior margin of the Falx cerebri in the midline. It empties into the **Sinus rectus (4)**, which runs backwards at the ridge of the Tentorium cerebelli and empties into the Confluens sinuum.

The Sinus rectus initially incorporates the **V. cerebri magna (vein of Galen, 10)**, which is formed below the Splenium corporis callosi from the **V. cerebri interna (11)** and the **V. basalis (12)**. The Confluens sinuum represents the confluence of the Sinus rectus and the Sinus sagittalis superior. From the Confluens sinuum the venous blood drains primarily through the **Sinus transversi (5)**. The Sinus transversi runs rostrally along the lateral border of the Tentorium cerebelli to the base of the petrous part of the temporal bone (➤ Chap. 7.2) and incorporates further along its course veins from the basal cerebral surface as well as cerebellar veins.

The **Sinus sigmoideus (6)** represents a continuation of the Sinus transversus. It arches in an S-shape in the Sulcus sinus sigmoidei towards the Foramen jugulare. Here it empties into the **V. jugularis interna (13)**.

The **Sinus occipitalis (7)** represents a further drainage route from the Confluens sinuum, which descends to the Foramen magnum and there empties via the Sinus marginalis (not shown) into the V. jugularis interna.

Ventral group of the Sinus durae matris

The ventral group consists of:

- **Sinus cavernosus (14)**
- **Sinus sphenoparietalis (15)**
- **Sinus petrosus superior (16)**
- **Sinus petrosus inferior** (not shown)

The sinuses of the ventral group empties into the **Sinus cavernosus (14)**. It lies paired in the area of the Sella turcica (➤ Chap. 7.2). The A. carotis interna and the N. abducens run through it. Inside its walls are the Nn. oculomotorius (N. III), trochlearis (N. IV) and ophthalmicus (N. V/1). Both of the Sinus cavernosi are connected to each other, so that it forms a ring around the pituitary gland. The Sinus cavernosus incorporates the **V. ophthalmica (17)** from the orbita. The venous sinuses of the brain are connected to the veins of the head via the V. ophthalmica; via the **V. angularis (18)** of the **V. facialis (19)**, as well as via the **Plexus pterygoideus (20)**.

The **Sinus sphenoparietalis (15)** also empties into the Sinus cavernosus.

From the Sinus cavernosus the blood flows via the **Sinus petrosus superior (16)** along the upper side of the petrous part of the temporal bone to the Sinus sigmoideus. The Sinus petrosus superior thus connects the ventral and dorsal groups of the Sinus durae matris.

> **Note**
>
> The venous blood of the brain is drained via the Sinus durae matris, valveless sinuses in the duplicatures of the dura mater, and finally flows into the V. jugularis interna.

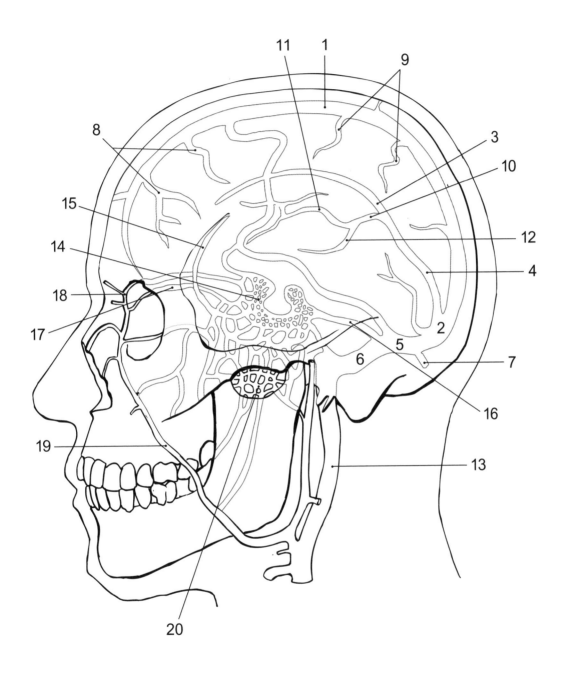

Abb. 9.9

191

9.9 The inner cerebrospinal fluid spaces

The brain and the spine are completely surrounded by a fluid, the **cerebrospinal fluid**. The fluid is here contained in the **subarachnoid space** between the meninges, more specifically between the Arachnoidea and the Pia mater.

There are also cavities filled with cerebrospinal fluid (CSF) in the central nervous system (CNS). The CNS is formed embryonically from the **neural tube.** Thereby, from the walls of the neural tube, the various sections of the CNS are formed, and from its lumen, the **inner cerebrospinal fluid spaces**.

- Both the **lateral ventricles** are situated in the **telencephalon.** They are structured as follows: In the frontal lobe is the **anterior horn (Cornu frontale, 1a),** in the parietal lobe is the **Pars centralis (1b),** in the temporal lobe is the **temporal horn (Cornu temporale, 1c)** and in the occipital lobe is the **occipital horn (Cornu occipitale, 1d).**

- Because all inner CSF spaces are formed from the lumen of the neural tube, they are all connected to each other. The **IIIrd ventricle (3),** the CSF space of the **diencephalon,** is reached via the **Foramina interventricularia (2).** Its lateral border is formed by the thalamus and the hypothalamus. The thalami on both sides are in contact with each other in the **Adhaesio interthalamica,** whereby a rounded recess is formed **(3a).** The IIIrd ventricle shows four small extensions. The **Recessus infundibuli (3b)** of the pituitary stalk, and the **Recessus supraopticus (3c)** towards the optic chiasm, as well as the **Recessus suprapinealis (3d)** and **pinealis (3e)** in the area of the epiphysis can be seen the optic chiasm.

- In the **mesencephalon,** the CSF space becomes constricted to form the **Aquaeductus mesencephali (4).**

- Via it, the IIIrd ventricle is in contact with the CSF space of the **hindbrain, the IVth ventricle (5).** It is bounded by the **cerebellum (6)** and the **brainstem (7).** In the IVth ventricle on both sides is the **Recessus lateralis (5a),** which respectively lead to the **Apertura lateralis (5b).** The unpaired **Apertura mediana (8)** point in the direction of the cerebellum. The CSF spaces are in contact with the subarachnoid space via these openings.

- Caudally, the IVth ventricle continues into the **central canal (9)** of the **spinal cord**.

The CSF fluid is formed continuously in the **Plexus choroideus** of the inner CSF spaces. The **Plexus choroideus** is present on the floor of the **Pars centralis (1b)** as well as on the roof of the **temporal horn (1c)** of the lateral ventricles, runs through the **Foramina interventricularia (2)** and then lies on the roof of the **IIIrd ventricle (3).** Also on the roof of the **IVth ventricle (5)** there is a Plexus choroideus, which continues into the **Recessus lateralis (5a)** and protrudes into the subarachnoid space via the **Apertura lateralis (5b).**

Reabsorption of the fluid takes place in the lymph vessels at the exit points of the spinal nerves and via the arachnoidal villi in the Sinus durae matris.

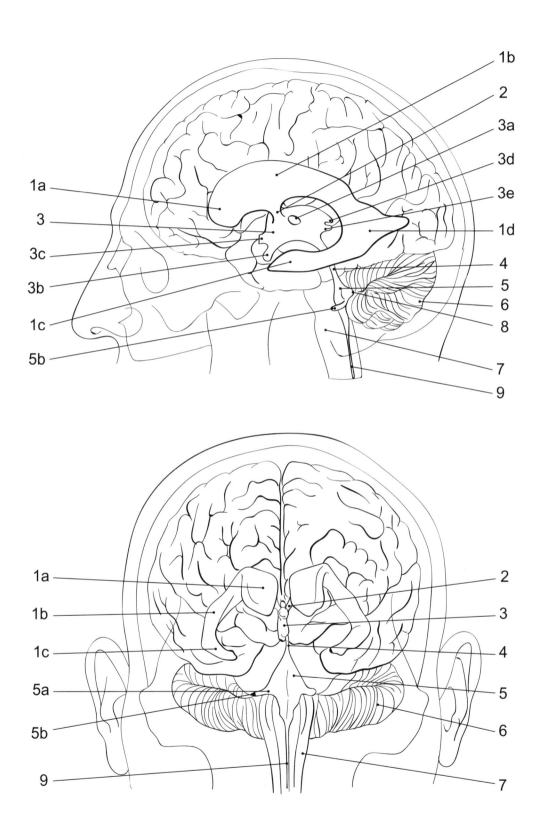

Abb. 9.10

193

9.10 Frontal section of the brain I

Structures in the depths of the brain can be seen in a series of frontal sections. With each sectional plane, different structures become visible. In the illustration, the incision has been made closely behind the Genu corporis callosi (see orientation sketch).

With an initial superficial view of the brain, it is possible to orientate oneself with familiar structures. The **Lobus frontalis (A1–3)** with its **Gyri frontales superior (A1)**, **medius (A2)** und **inferior (A3)** is visible, as well as the rostral pole of the **Lobus temporalis (B)**. Both lobes are separated from each other by the **Sulcus lateralis (1)**.

On the surface it is now also possible to discern the **grey matter of the cerebral cortex (2)** consisting primarily of neural cells, and the underlying **white matter (3)**. From above, the **Fissura longitudinalis cerebri (4)** cuts in deeply and separates both of the cerebral hemispheres from each other. The biggest commissure, the **Corpus callosum (5a and b),** is affected in two places (see orientation sketch): one is the **truncus (5a)** and the other the **rostrum (5b)**.

In the depths of the brain, two cavities can be seen, the **lateral ventricles (Ventriculi laterales, 6)**, here in the area of their anterior horns (Cornua anteriora). They represent the inner CSF spaces of the telencephalon and are separated from each other by the **Septum pellucidum (7)** which lies below the Corpus callosum.

It is also noticeable that grey matter is present in the depths of the telencephalon and not only on the cerebral cortex. Visible are sections of the **Caput nuclei caudati (8)** on the floor and in the lateral wall of the Ventriculus lateralis, and of the **putamen (9)**. Both structures are seen as part of the basal ganglia. They are connected to each other by bridges of grey matter, which gives them a stripy appearance. Both together are therefore described as **Corpus striatum**.

The **Capsula interna (10)** lies between the bridges of grey matter. It is formed by projection tracts, which come from the caudal brain areas and run in between the basal ganglia through to the cerebral cortex or in the opposite direction.

Clinical remarks

To assess illnesses and injuries to the brain, **Computed tomography (CT scan)** and **magnetic resonance imaging (MRI scan)** is used. This gives precise information on the anatomical cross-sections.

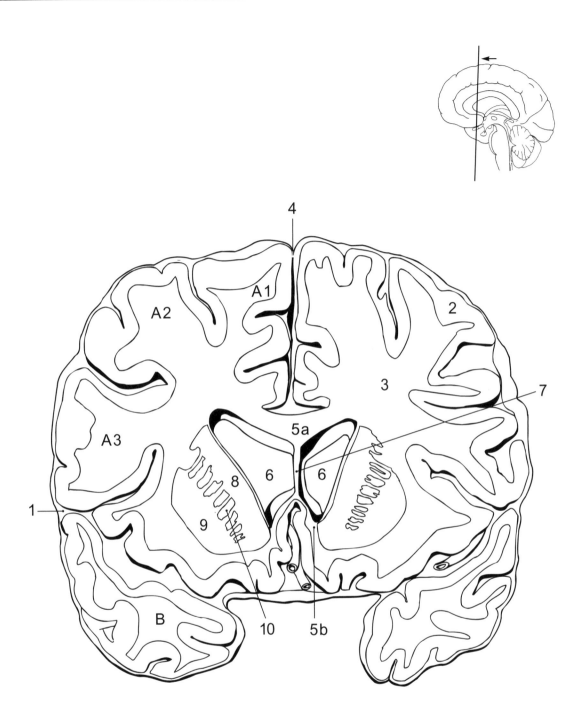

Abb. 9.11

9.11 Frontal section of the brain II

This frontal section was made at the level of the **pituitary gland (1)** and just behind the **Commissura anterior (2)** (see orientation sketch). The structures which are already familiar are:

- **Lobus frontalis (A1–3)** with the **Gyri frontales superior (A1), medius (A2)** and **inferior (A3)**
- **Lobus temporalis (B1–3)** with the **Gyri temporales superior (B1), medius (B2)** and **inferior (B3)**
- **Gyri occipitotemporales laterales (3), mediales (4)** and **Gyrus parahippocampalis (5)**,
- **Truncus corporis callosi (6)**
- **Fissura longitudinalis cerebri (7)** and **Sulcus lateralis (8)**

The gyri of the brain are present in the depths of the **Sulcus lateralis**, hidden in the lateral view by the frontal and parietal lobes. These gyri are the **Gyri insulae (9)**.

In the area of the **basal ganglia**, the already familiar sections of the **Caput nuclei caudati (10)** and of the **putamen (11)** are visible, as well as the **Capsula interna (12)** which runs between them. Between the Gyri insulae and the putamen, a narrow strip of grey matter can now also be seen, the **claustrum (13)**.

Medial to the **putamen (11)** a further nuclear area can be discerned, the **Globus pallidus (14)**, from which it is possible to differentiate a **lateral (14a)** and a **medial (14b) part**.

With the **claustrum (13)**, two narrow strips of white matter are separated between the Gyri insulae and the claustrum as well as between the claustrum and the putamen:

- **Capsula extrema (15)**
- **Capsula externa (16)**

On the lower margin of the **Septum pellucidum (17)** and medial of the Capsula interna it is possible to see sections of the **corpus (18a)** and the **columns (18b)** of the **fornix (18)**, a projection tract which connects the Corpora mammillaria of the diencephalon with the hippocampus (➤ Chap. 9.12).

The inner CSF space of the diencephalon is visible (the **3rd ventricle (Ventriculus tertius, 19)** below the fornix (18). In this sectional plane, the lateral ventricle and the 3rd ventricle are closely in contact with each other via the **Foramina interventricularia (20)** behind the fornix. The wall of the 3rd ventricle forms the **hypothalamus (21)**. The **pituitary stalk (22)** exits basally from here. Below the hypothalamus is the **Tractus opticus (23)**, a part of the visual pathway which belongs to the diencephalon.

In the temporal lobe (Lobus temporalis) a further section of the lateral ventricle can be seen, extending into the temporal lobe, on an archshaped course with its **Cornu inferius (24)**. Similarly, the drawn-out **tail** of the **caudate nucleus (Cauda nuclei caudati, 25)** is shaped like a comet, which comes to rest here in the roof of the Cornu inferius.

Next to the Cornu inferius, another nuclear area, the **Corpus amygdaloideum (26)**, can be seen in this sectional plane.

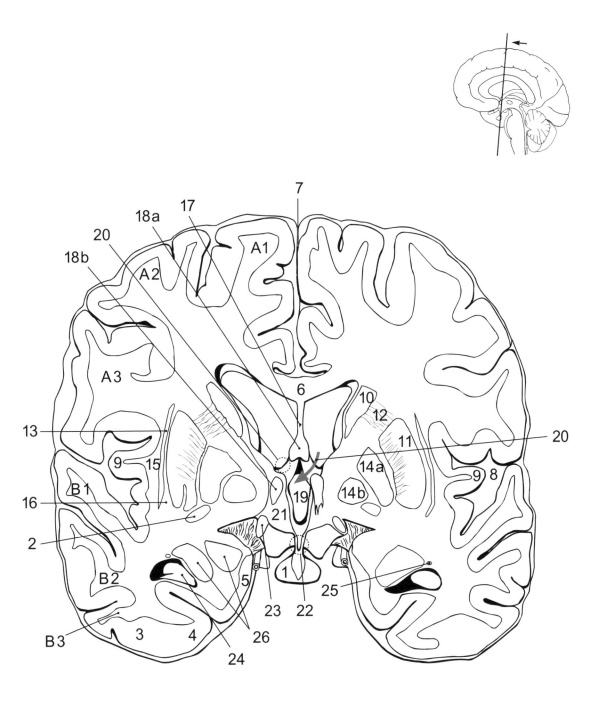

Abb. 9.12

197

9.12 Frontal section of the brain III

The sectional plane at the level of the Corpora mammillaria shows the **pons (1)** as well as the gyri in the frontal and temporal lobes, already visible in the previous section (see orientation sketch).

The **Ventriculus lateralis (2)** is shown here in its Pars centralis. On its floor it is possible to see the **Plexus choroideus ventriculi lateralis (3)**, where cerebrospinal fluid is formed.

The Plexus choroidei of the lateral ventricles are in contact with the **Tela choroidea (4)** in the roof of the **Ventriculus tertius (5)** at the level of the Foramina interventricularia (➤ Chap. 9.11). **Truncus corporis callosi (6)** is in the roof of the lateral ventricles also and **Corpora nuclei caudati (7)** in its lateral wall.

The **Septum pellucidum (8)** stretches out below the Corpus callosum and below that the **Corpus fornicis (9)**. In the wall of the 3rd ventricle lies the **thalamus (10)** which belongs to the diencephalon. The **Corpora mammillaria (11)** are on the floor of the 3rd ventricle.

In the area of the basal ganglia are the **claustrum (12)**, the **putamen (13)**, the **Globus pallidus (14)** and the **nucleus caudate (7),** as well as the white matter which lies between (**Capsula extrema, 15, externa, 16,** and **interna, 17**).

The **insular cortex (Gyri insulae, 19)** are in the depths of the **Sulcus lateralis (18).** The **Cornu inferius (20)** of the lateral ventricle can now be seen more clearly in the area of the Lobus temporalis. In its roof lies the **Cauda nuclei caudati (21)**. From medial, the **hippocampus (22)** protrudes in the lumen of the Cornu inferius. Because of its spirally winding structure, this cerebral cortex area is also called the Cornu ammonis. Above the Cornu inferius lies the **Corpus amygdaloideum (23)**.

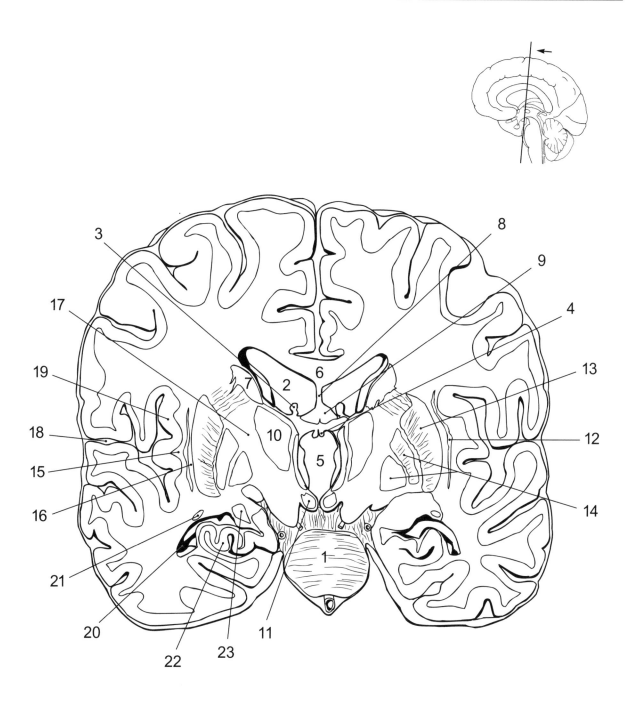

Abb. 9.13

199

9.13 Frontal section of the brain IV

This frontal section lies at the level of the **Glandula pinealis (epiphysis, 1)** and the **4th ventricle (Ventriculus quartus, 2)**. The dorsal sectional surface (see orientation sketch) shows the **Splenium corporis callosi (3)**, the **cerebellum (4)** and the **Medulla oblongata (myelencephalon, 5)**.

In the area of the Cortex cerebri, the **Gyri postcentralis (6), parietalis inferior (7)** and **supramarginalis (8)** are now also seen.

Laterally of the **Splenium corporis callosi (3)** lies the **Pars centralis of the Ventriculus lateralis (9)** with the **Plexus choroideus (10)**. The Plexus choroideus extends into the **Cornu inferius (11)** to the lateral ventricle. It is possible to see the **Crura fornicis (12)**, which also lies laterally of the splenium. Here they turn away from the midline and run in an arch to the **hippocampus (13)**.

Below the splenium, the **Glandula pinealis (epiphysis, 1)** has been truncated. The outer surface of the brain can be seen in the area of the epiphysis. The **Pulvinar thalami (14)** can here be seen showing its surface (left) and truncated (right). The **Colliculi superiores (15)** and **inferiores (16)** of the Tectum mesencephali are visible from dorsal below the epiphysis.

The **cerebellum (4)** is in contact with the brainstem via the **Pedunculi cerebellares superior (17), medius (18)** and **inferior (19)**. Besides the **cerebellar hemispheres (4a)**, it is possible to see the **Vermis cerebelli (4b)**, also situated in the midline. Between the cerebellum and the brainstem, the CSF space of the rhombencephalon, the **4th ventricle (2),** is truncated.

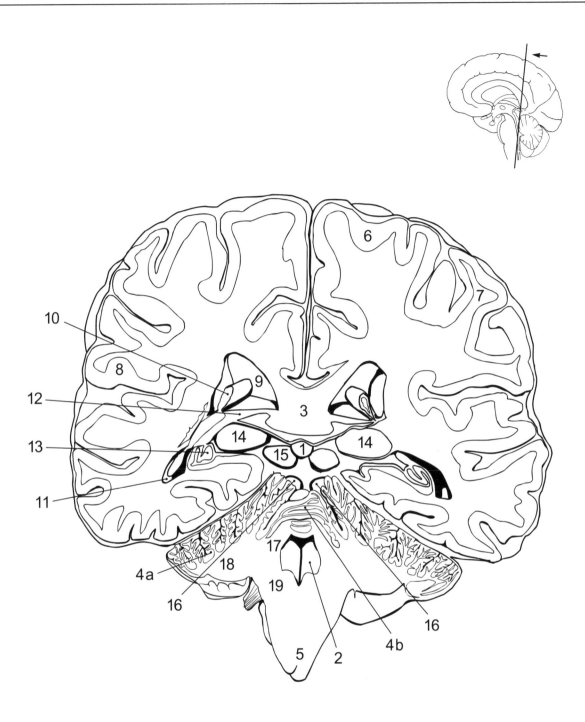

Abb. 9.14

9.14 Horizontal section of the brain

In the horizontal section through the brain, some topographical links of the deep cranial areas are more marked than in the frontal section. This horizontal section was made at the level of the **rostrum (1)** of the corpus callosum and directly underneath the **splenium**.

With an initial orientation by looking at the surface structures, the deeply penetrating **Sulcus lateralis (2)** and the **insula (3)** become clear. In the depths, nuclei of the **basal ganglia** border the insular cortex. From the outside to the inside are the:

- **Claustrum (4)**
- **Putamen (5)**
- **Globus pallidum (6)**

Further medially, the **Capsula interna** adjoins with its **anterior (7a)** und **posterior (7b) limb** and the **genu (7c)** an. Through it, descending motor and ascending sensory tracts run from and/ or to the cortex. Further medially, the anterior limb of the Capsula interna is bounded by the **Caput nuclei caudati (8)**, which can here be seen in the wall of the anterior horn of the **lateral ventricle (9)**. The medial border of the posterior limb of the Capsula interna forms the **thalamus (10),** in which almost all afferent, sensory tracts are crossed.

Of the **ventricle system,** the **third ventricle (11)** as well as the **occipital horns (12)** of the lateral ventricles can be seen. In them is a part of the **Plexus choroideus (13),** one of the places where fluid is formed. Ventrally of the third ventricle there are two small, rounded sections on the **Columna fornicis (14a).** The **fornix** is a projection tract which runs in the shape of an arch from the diencephalon to the hippocampus. Correspondingly, there is a second section through the **Fimbria hippocampi (14b)** on the medial edge of the occipital horn of the lateral ventricle. Dorsally of the third ventricle lies the **Corpus pineale (15),** a structure of the diencephalon, which helps to regulate the day-night rhythm.

In the area of the occipital lobe – around the deeply penetrating **Sulcus calcarinus (16)** – is the **visual cortex (17).** Protruding from the posterior limb of the Capsula interna, the **Radiatio optica (18)** can be seen macroscopically. In it, the **visual pathway** runs from the thalamus to the visual cortex.

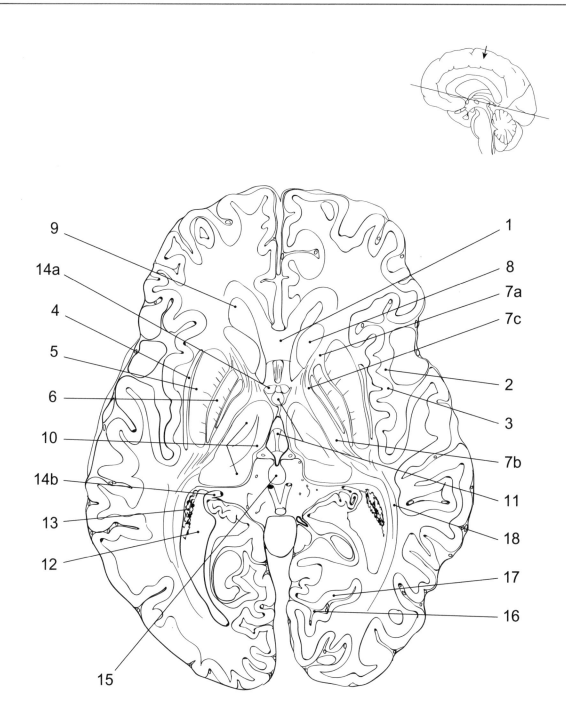

9

14a

4

5

6

10

14b

13

12

15

1

8

7a

7c

2

3

7b

11

18

17

16

Abb. 9.15

203

9.15 Vertebral canal, spinal cord and spinal nerves

The spinal column encompasses the **vertebral canal (Canalis vertebralis, 1)**. The vertebral canal contains the **spinal cord (A1 and 2)**, from which the **spinal nerves** originate.

Vertebral canal   The **spinal cord (A1 and 2)** lies in the vertebral canal **(Canalis vertebralis, 1)**, which is formed by the successive **vertebrae (B1–6)**. The top illustration shows by way of example a vertebra with a **Corpus vertebrae (B1)**, the **Arcus vertebrae (B2)** as well as its processes, the **Processus transversi (B3)** , **spinosus (B4)** and **articulares superior (B5)** and **inferior (B6)**. The **Ligg. longitudinale anterius (2)** and **posterius (3)** run in front of and/or behind the vertebral body. Between the vertebral bodies lie the cartilaginous **Disci intervertebrales (intervertebral discs, 4)**.

Spinal cord   The bottom illustration of a spinal cord segment shows the superficially lying **white matter (A1)** of the spinal cord, which subdivides into an **anterolateral tract (A1.1)** and a **posterior funiculus (A1.2)**. The **grey matter (A2)** of the spinal cord lies in a butterfly shape in the depths. In it, a squat **Cornu anterius (anterior horn, A2.1)** and a narrower **Cornu posterius (occipital horn, A2.2)** can be differentiated. In the area of the anterolateral tract, the neural fibres leave the spinal column as **Radix anterior (5)**, while in the area of the occipital horn, neural fibres enter the spinal cord as **Radix posterior (6)**. These fibres represent somatosensory afferents, of which the neuronal cell bodies lie in the **Ganglion spinale (spinal ganglion, 7)**.

Spinal nerves   The Radices anterior and posterior of each spinal cord segment unite to become a **N. spinalis (spinal nerve, 8)**. Thereby altogether 31 spinal nerve pairs (8 Nn. cervicales, 12 Nn. thoracici, 5 Nn. lumbales, 5 Nn. sacrales, 1 N. coccygeus) are formed. In the area of the **Foramina intervertebralia (9)**, these divide into five branches:

- **R. anterior (10)**
- **R. posterior (11)**
- **R. meningeus recurrens (12)**
- **Rr. communicantes albus (13)** and **griseus (14)**

The Rr. communicantes connect the spinal nerves with the **Truncus sympathicus (sympathetic trunk, 15)**, which lies ventrally on the vertebral bodies.

Vessel supply of the spinal cord   The spinal cord is supplied from the **A. spinalis anterior (16)** and both of the **Aa. spinales posteriores (17)** . They exit from the A. vertebralis intracranially and then run caudally in the Fissura mediana anterior and/or along the Sulcus posterolateralis. The caudal spinal cord (especially in the thickened Intumescentia lumbosacralis, rich in neural cells) receives from the A. lumbales or directly from the Aorta abdominalis via the radicular arteries an additional and significant inflow. The biggest of these radicular arteries is the **A. radicularis magna (Adamkiewicz artery, 18)**.

> **Note**
>
> **Branches of the spinal nerves**
> - R. anterior **(10)**
> - R. posterior **(11)**
> - R. meningeus recurrens **(12)**
> - Rr. communicantes albus **(13)** and griseus **(14)**

> **Clinical remarks**
>
> With degenerative changes in the Disci intervertebrales, its gelatinous Nucleus pulposus can prolapse and compress the spinal nerve or its roots in the area of the Foramen intervertebrale **(spinal disk herniation)**. Besides pain, segmental loss of sensory and motor function can result.

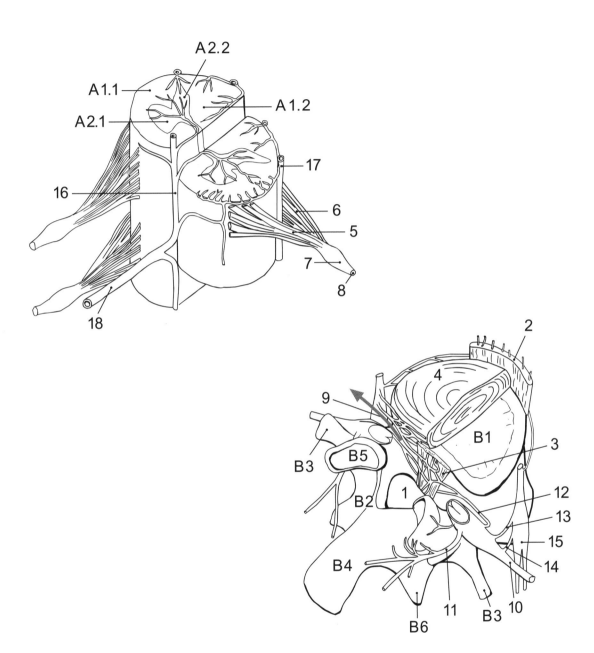

Abb. 9.16

205

Index

Index English (Latin)

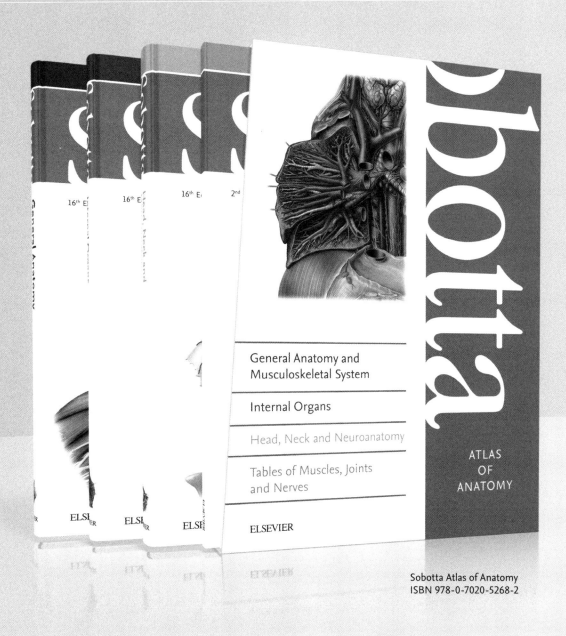
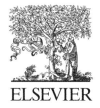

Sobotta Anatomy Textbook

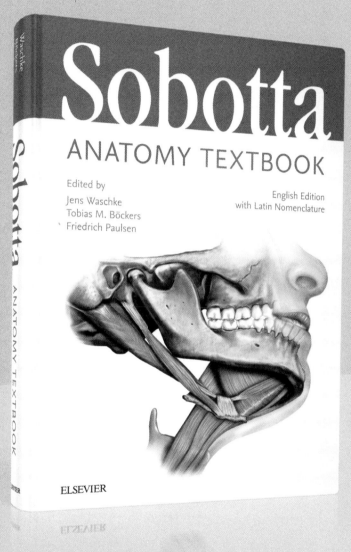

Sobotta Anatomy Textbook
ISBN 978-0-7020-6760-0

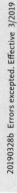
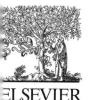

ELSEVIER

These and many other titles are available at local bookshops,
as well as at **shop.elsevier.com**, which also gives the current prices

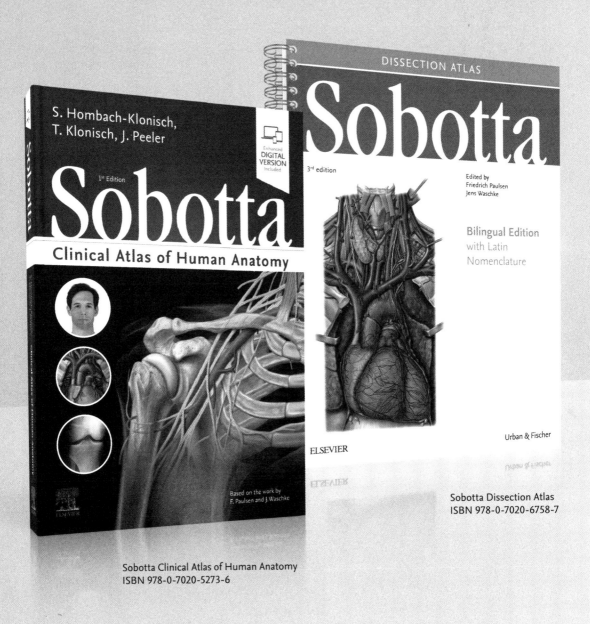
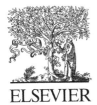